La Clínica

Literature and Medicine Series

STATEMENT OF PURPOSE: The art of writing and the science of medicine offer very different approaches to some of the most intense and mysterious human experiences. The Literature and Medicine series, jointly sponsored by the University of New Mexico Press and the University of New Mexico's Health Sciences Center, brings together these two ways of understanding. Comprising fiction and creative nonfiction, the series showcases stories that explore the nature of health and healing and the texture of the experience of illness.

ADVISORY EDITORS: Elizabeth Hadas, Frank Huyler, M.D., and David P. Sklar, M.D.

La Clínica

A Doctor's Journey Across Borders

David P. Sklar

UNIVERSITY OF NEW MEXICO PRESS •≈• ALBUQUERQUE

Library of Congress Cataloging-in-Publication Data

Sklar, David P.
La clinica : a doctor's journey across borders /
David P. Sklar.
      p. cm. — (Literature and Medicine Series)
ISBN 978-0-8263-4524-0 (cloth : alk. paper)
1. Sklar, David P.
2. Emergency physicians—New Mexico—Albuquerque—Biography.
3. Emergency physicians—Mexico—Biography.
4. Clinics—Mexico.
5. Rural health services—Mexico.
I. Title.
RA975.5.E5.S55 2008
610.92—dc22
   [B]
2008015002

Book design and type composition by Melissa Tandysh

Composed in 11/14 Warnock Pro

Display type is Brioso Pro Semibold

To my parents, Selma and Albert Sklar;

my sister Diane;

and my brothers, Mark and Ron.

PREFACE

Stories that involve relationships between physicians and patients run the risk of either violating the privacy and confidentiality of the relationship or becoming so altered through efforts to disguise identities as to border on fiction. I have attempted to protect identities by changing names and altering characteristics while maintaining the key elements of the relationships and events. In some cases, temporal sequences were altered to maintain the narrative flow of a story that unfolded over twenty-five years.

Some of the topics raised in this book may be difficult for some readers. However, I hope the book will deepen our understanding of the complex motives and consequences inherent in helping relationships, whether in a foreign place or in our own home communities.

ACKNOWLEDGMENTS

I had the good fortune to be the recipient of help from many people during the development of this book. Frank Huyler—first my student, then my colleague, and then my mentor—provided invaluable advice and unswerving encouragement. Julie Reichert read many drafts of the manuscript and offered helpful advice through all phases of the book's evolution. I would also like to thank friends and family who provided assistance and encouragement—Della, Dan, Lisa, Ariel, Ethan, Nyika, Jos, and Moshe. University of New Mexico Press former editor Beth Hadas and present editor Clark Whitehorn both provided encouragement and advice.

I would like to particularly thank my life partner, Deborah Helitzer, for her steadfast support and loving encouragement.

Prologue

WE HOISTED THE BODIES ONTO GURNEYS AND CUT THE blood-drenched clothes from their heaving limbs, necks, and chests— John Does 1, 2, and 3, because we didn't know their names. Paramedics, holding bottles of clear intravenous fluid, described what happened— a gang fight with knives and baseball bats. Blood pooled on the floor. Nurses and paramedics ran into the room and out of the room, bumping into each other, eyes jumping from body to floor and back. An intern kept checking for pulses in the arms and neck and legs, looking up at me as the paramedics began to do CPR. I stood at the head of the bed, smelling the sweat and blood, checking the laryngoscope bulb, looking down at the long face and the body of John Doe 1.

He had large protruding ears and broad muscular shoulders that contrasted with the delicate face of a crying Jesus tattooed on his chest. A single tear hung suspended near his left nipple. His calloused hands had probably carried heavy boards and beams for houses. His eyes stared up at the ceiling. When the paramedics began CPR, I knew it was probably hopeless. I said, "Open him," and the surgery resident cut through the face of Jesus down to the lungs and heart. Blood spilled out all over the gurney, gushing from the hole in the heart.

"Stop," I said. "He's dead." I watched the heart manage an occasional, ineffective beat. "Let's move on to the next one."

John Doe 2 had buckteeth with braces. His parents had spent thousands of dollars on his mouth. He died slowly as we X-rayed his chest, probed the wound under his rib cage, and inserted tubes and catheters in every place we imagined it might help. His blood pressure had dropped suddenly when he returned from X-ray, and we were trying to figure out what the knife had cut.

"Call the OR," I said, scanning the room for the surgeon. And the surgeons took him up, but he died in the operating room of a cut vena cava.

John Doe 3 survived. He cried for his mother as we stuck needles into his veins. He had a stab wound through a spider web tattooed on his shoulder. He was fourteen or maybe fifteen, and he watched his friends die on the gurneys next to him. I looked at his eyes as they darted about. "You'll be OK," I said.

The nurses were calling to me. "David—Dr. Sklar—what should we do about John Doe 1?"

"Put his body in the hall," I said.

"What about John Doe 2? They brought his body back from the OR."

"In the hallway too, next to John Doe 1."

As they called my name, it reminded me of Mexico, of the first time a villager had called my name to help someone sick, someone dying.

"David," they would whisper at my window at night. "*Por favor*, David," they'd say and then knock lightly and insistently to waken me. Even though I was only twenty-two years old and was not yet a doctor, and even though I barely understood their language, they would come to my window in the middle of the night.

And I'd dress and stumble over the uneven rocks of the unlit street to an adobe house with a single lantern illuminating a feverish patient lying on a burlap cot in the darkest corner of the room. I'd smell the strange pungent herbs and oils covering a place where the pain resided, usually the middle of the belly, or under a breast.

After a while they'd whisper my name again. "David, David, is there no medicine for this?"

And I'd have to walk back across the village to the clinic to find something that might help.

Now, I walked out to the ambulance parking lot, following the nurses who needed a smoking break. John Doe 3 had been rolled down a corridor to the intensive care unit, and for a moment we were free. The janitor was already mopping up the floor, making the blood disappear, but now he stopped and followed us out, along with the two interns and a security guard. One of the interns fashioned a ball out of Kerlix bandage and white adhesive tape. The security guard rigged up some lighting for us, and the janitor unscrewed a broom handle so they could play stickball. I watched from the corner with the nurses, and we all inhaled the cool evening air and cigarette smoke.

The nurses looked at me suspiciously, expecting me to end this break and get everyone back to work. They knew there were patients waiting to be seen, and as the attending, I was ultimately responsible and could not condone any laziness. But I also knew that I could only push so far, that we all had a breaking point, and I felt we were close to it now. Even me.

I usually tried to keep my personal problems away from work, but tonight I was worn out. I had squeezed the last ounce of energy from my muscles, the last idea from my brain, and I felt drained. My wife had just moved out of our house and taken some of the furniture, and after work I'd return to a house without chairs or couches, without music, without lamps. But at least there was a bed, and I would dive under the covers, close the curtains, and pull the phone out of its jack in hopes of a good sleep. I needed a good sleep.

So when the nurses asked me how I was doing, how things were at home, I told them.

At first they stood, their mouths frozen to their cigarettes, eyes wide. And then I saw their arms open, and each one hugged me, pulled me close, blew cigarette breath into my face, and told me I'd be OK, that it had happened to each of them, that men were assholes—except for me.

As the interns played stickball, I walked away into the outfield and looked up into the sky. The same stars were all still there, just like every night.

When relatives or friends of the sick would come for me in Mexico, I'd gaze at the stars as I walked out of my house. In the village, without any electricity, the sky teemed with stars, and they filled up more of the blackness.

In those days, I carried with me a bag of equipment, a light, some pills, and a conviction that, whatever the gaps in my knowledge, I was better than nothing; I could make a difference. Now I wondered what had made me so sure and why I hadn't questioned myself— questioned all of us there—for pretending to know more or be more than we were.

Now as I walked out into the hospital parking lot, the blackness in the sky between the stars seemed to be expanding as my own doubts about myself grew. I had just watched two young men die. I didn't even know their names. I had their blood all over me—sticky red paint blotting out the stars, blotting out my marriage, my life. Why did I choose this life where I had to face death every day and wash the blood from my clothes? Was it time to give it up, let go, find something else to do?

And that was when I decided to retrace my path to the village where my medical career had begun, to the people and their stories that had inspired me to be not only a doctor, but also a good husband and father. The village and the clinic had been my engine all these years, powering me forward with a vision of why my life made sense and a certainty of its basic goodness. In the village the needs were obvious. If you worked hard enough, the dying might live, the suffering might be relieved, and you could feel good about your part in it. The clinic was a reminder of what we could do with effort and perseverance. But now I felt adrift, exhausted, and full of doubt. I began to think about all the bits of information that had accumulated over the years to contradict that vision. Complaints—about medical mistakes, long waits for care, and ineffective treatments—sat in a pile on my desk. And the love of my wife, which had coursed through me like the blood in my veins, had now been drained away. I wanted to discover what led me to make the choices that were now causing so much pain and to determine whether my image of the village, the clinic, and the relationships with the people there was based upon real memories or fantasies. Maybe that would help me discern the next step away from the fog enveloping me.

I heard the Kerlix-taped ball land a few feet away and picked it up. It glistened, white against the blackness of the asphalt. I squeezed it in my hand as I passed the interns, and they knew without my speaking, that it was time to go back to work.

Chapter One

MY PEN PAUSED ON THE WORD *PAIN*. "THIS IS A SEVENTY-five-year-old man with a chief complaint of chest pain." The pen drifted downward across the chart, as if it were a mountain climber sliding down a glacier, and finally dropped off into my lap causing me to startle, open my eyes, and realize I had fallen asleep. I looked up at the clock: 7:55 a.m. My relief would be here in a few minutes. I could coast and do nothing for the next five minutes and congratulate myself that I had made it through another night shift. My body ached, and my feet throbbed from the constant standing and walking. My back hurt from bending over and suturing a man's bleeding eyebrow. Someone had hit him with a bottle at the Blue Spruce, one of Albuquerque's most violent bars. My eyes were blurry, barely able to focus on the chart and the triage note. My stomach had cramps, which usually signaled diarrhea at the end of a shift.

"Hey, you look wiped out," said Rick, my replacement. Rick had been working in emergency medicine for close to twenty years. We had been residents together even before we worked in the emergency department. He made a point of stating the obvious, as if he were jotting down a data point in a research study. If we walked by a pale, lifeless body that had bled to death, he would say, "That guy looks bad." Or he would say, "Odor of alcohol on his breath," about a patient who was unconscious and reeking of alcohol. So when he said I looked wiped out, I realized I must look really exhausted.

"Yeah, it was one of those nights," I said.

"Well, better you than me." He laughed.

"Yeah, there was a gang fight. Two kids died from stabbings. There was blood everywhere; it was a mess," I said.

"Guns are cleaner," he said. Rick had straight brown hair combed back, thick glasses with wire rims, and a gray-brown beard, which often caught bits of food and ice cream. He always wore a tie and white shirt under his white coat and kept his black shoes shined. "We should hand out guns to all the gang kids and let them get it over with all at one time. Problem is, they are so stupid they'd probably miss."

"Rick, isn't that a little racist?" I said.

"It's not. I'm not saying that they are Mexicans or Indians or blacks or whites. It doesn't matter. But they're all stupid. They can't read. They knock up their thirteen-year-old girlfriends just to show off. And they knife each other because one guy stares at another through a car window and twists his finger wrong."

"I'm too tired to get into it with you now, but you know it's not that they are stupid or lazy. It's about not having a dad in the house, no jobs, and drugs on every corner. How can you come in here every day and take care of them if you hate them so much?" I asked.

"It's like veterinary medicine. You just have to watch out for the teeth and claws. It's like a zoo. Don't you like watching the chimpanzees and the polar bears and the tigers? I like going to the zoo," he said, laughing.

We walked around the emergency department and went from bed to bed. "Bed 1 is a forty-two-year-old woman with possible appendicitis who is waiting to go to the OR. Check and make sure the surgeons don't forget about her. Bed 2 is a thirty-year-old woman with pancreatitis. Her amylase is 4,000, and her calcium is 7.9. She's admitted to medicine."

"How long has she been waiting?" he asked.

"Just a few hours," I said, and he nodded.

"I'm sick of all these patients waiting for beds," he said. "I don't want to know about anyone who has already been admitted."

"But, Rick, what if something happens, and a nurse comes to you with a request? Don't you want to have a note written down so you can do something?"

"No," he said. "It's not my problem. I'd rather not know about it. It's like those starving children in Africa. When you see pictures of them, you feel bad and want to send money. So if you don't see the pictures, it's better. I don't want to know about the admitted patients."

"OK," I said. "That will shorten rounds and I'll get home sooner."

"Hey, I hope this isn't going to affect my evaluation," he said, laughing. "Aren't we doing one of those this week? I got to be careful what I say to the chairman."

"Rick, your evaluation will be based on the forms filled out by the residents and nurses. By the time we meet, I won't even remember we had this conversation. My mind goes blank after a night shift."

"Yeah, you're too old for them," he said.

"Well you're older than I am," I said. We completed rounds, skipping over the admitted patients.

I drove home in a daze. I closed my eyes at a red light and began to dream. I woke up with a start as the car behind me honked to alert me to the green light.

When I got to my house, the dog was waiting. He barked and jumped up on my legs as I stepped from the car, almost knocking me down.

"Down, Chamisa," I said, and I let the dog into the house with me.

I headed straight for the bedroom. Boxes packed with pictures and pottery lined the hallway, and lamps were missing. Bookcases were empty. "What is she doing?" I thought to myself. Even with this evidence that Laura had moved out and had packed up a few remaining objects, I still could not believe it. And then I remembered that she had told me she was going to come over in the morning and pack up more boxes.

"Maybe if I'm asleep, I won't have to talk to her," I thought.

The bedroom felt cold and lonely. The bed lay unmade in the center of the room, sheets bundled together with a blue blanket twisted inside like pastry filling. Nails dotted the walls where pictures had hung. A lamp sat on the floor rather than on the side table where it had been before, and the side table was gone. I spread out the sheets and blanket and plunged under them as if I were diving deep under the water, and immediately I began to imagine fish and coral and seahorses floating up toward me. When I was exhausted after a night shift, I would often feel my mind racing, even as the rest of my body tried to shut down. The key was to find an image that could slow my mind and erase the patients, the lab tests, the conversations with my wife—the problems that would only prevent me from sleeping as I jumped from issue to issue. And so I thought of tropical fish floating over black coral: blue fish with yellow stripes, black-and-white zebra fish, red groupers, black and gray stingrays, conch shells, sea horses, and starfish.

And then a thought, an intrusion into the peaceful ocean. My mind got caught on a problem that had been lurking in a corner of my memory: Laura needed money for the apartment she was renting. We needed to take it out of our bank account that had been meant for the children's education. How would we ever pay for college? The kids would have to go to trade school or become garbage collectors. Until I banished these crazy thoughts and replaced them with better memories, I would be spinning around faster and faster with fear.

I thought of my first girlfriend, Ann, who kissed me on a cold summer night in Maine as I sat behind the steering wheel after our first date and tried to figure out how to get my arms around her and not tangled up in the steering wheel. I was sixteen, and she was fourteen, with beautiful long legs, straight blond hair, and a sharp turned-up nose. I thought about how we had never slept together, about how it might have been. And how my fantasy about it had kept her image alive and intriguing for all these years. I felt my breathing slow, and my body began to relax.

Before I could drift off to sleep, another intrusion awakened my mind. My muscles tightened, and my heart sped up. I found myself thinking about Rick, what a jerk he was, how he did not care about the patients or the nurses, what I would do about it when I performed his evaluation, and whether anyone would die because he didn't want to listen to me during check-out. The woman with appendicitis could die if Rick didn't follow up and get the surgeons down to take her to the operating room. Of course, if she were upstairs in the hospital, we wouldn't even know about any of this. I wondered if I should get out of bed and call him. Now that I was worried about it, I might never fall asleep until I called him.

I tried to let it go. I thought about my family. My grandfather, Israel Sklar, had grown up in Russia and stowed away on a ship to come to the United States when he was seventeen. He founded the family business, Sklar Oil Company, by saving his money, buying an old oil truck, and delivering heating oil to homes of other Yiddish-speaking immigrants. When they could not pay, he would take credit. He had a completely bald head perched upon a large, round body, and he spoke English with a strong Yiddish accent. One day after I had practiced my Hebrew prayers with the rabbi for my upcoming Bar Mitzvah, I ran into him at the synagogue. He was vice president of the congregation and prayed at the temple every day.

"Hi, Gran'pa," I said.

"Hi, Davidil," he said. "So, *vus is nu?*"

"Well Gran'pa," I said. "I was thinking of becoming a rabbi." I expected him to smile, maybe even hug me, but instead, he frowned.

"You're a smart boy," he said. "Be a doctor. Rabbis don't make money."

"But I'm studying all the prayers, and I like to study Torah. Don't you want me to be a rabbi?"

"Be a doctor," he said, dismissing me, his mind already full of other problems.

That was the first time I thought about becoming a doctor. But it had nothing to do with what a doctor did. It was only about pleasing my grandfather. Later, my mother told me she had always wanted to become a doctor, but her family was too poor. She grew up in the Depression with only her mother, grandmother, and aunt. Her father had died of tuberculosis when she was one, and the family had to live on her aunt's librarian salary. Since medical school was out of the question, my mother entered the state teacher's college, and then she met my dad, who had just returned from Germany, a World War II hero.

"I was in love," my mother would say, "and I wanted to be a doctor, not a teacher."

"But couldn't both of you have gone to college and worked part time?"

"No, everyone was starting families, and your grandfather needed help with the business. Before we knew it, we had three children and a house, and you can't go back from that."

"But are you happy?" I asked her.

"Sure, I am happy enough, and one day you will be able to do what I couldn't do. If you use the opportunity you have, you will make me happy." We had this conversation when I was twelve and my mother was still young. She had a habit of avoiding personal questions that might lead to issues she did not want to discuss. And she did not want to discuss whether she was happy. But in case I was wondering, I could solve the question by becoming a doctor, and then she would certainly be happy.

The thoughts of my family developed into another distraction. I thought of my parents and their wonderful marriage. I would be the first in the family to get divorced. I had never failed at anything before. Even in basketball, where my height of five feet seven inches was a disadvantage, I had practiced and practiced until I made the team. But now I was failing. I wondered how many other failures there were in my life: mistakes with patients, rejections of manuscripts from my research studies, memory lapses, and wrong dosages of digoxin. Did I give the wrong dose last night? My mind raced along, and I was wide awake again. I sighed. "Maybe I should take a sleeping pill," I thought. I hated to do it, because taking the pill dropped me into a deep, mindless coma, and I felt hung over when I awakened.

I tried one more time. I thought about that happy time in the Philippines, when I went there to be a volunteer teacher after two years at Stanford. I was tired of classes and studying. I wanted to experience the dialectical materialism and praxis of Marx, Marcuse, and Paul Baran—and figure out what I would do after I finished college. The thrill of co-ed dorms and drugs had worn thin, and I was ready to see another part of the world.

I arrived at a dense, green jungle in a tropical downpour. And I remember thinking, "This is so green, so different; it's another world." I walked and slid along a mud path to my cabin and spent most of my first day sleeping and listening to the rain. I was assigned English, history, and psychology as my courses to teach, and a sloping field to cultivate for vegetables that would feed the school for several months.

After a few weeks at the school, one of my students, Rudi, invited me to visit his family in their bamboo hut on the beach. "We're very poor," he said as we neared the hut, and I could see the embarrassment and anxiety in his eyes.

"It's OK," I said. "I don't care. I want to meet your family."

The house sat on poles that disappeared into the water. We walked across a bamboo bridge and slept on the floor, all in the same room, in a row like pastries. Rudi's father fished at night, using a lantern to attract the sparse marine life. He spent the entire night out, returning with one small bony fish, which Rudi's mother prepared for me.

She fried it in lard in a black pan over a fire in the back of the house. Everyone watched me eat and laughed as I tried to spoon in rice and fish with my right hand—without utensils—and spilled rice and fish on my stomach and the bamboo floor. "My mother says, 'How can he be so smart if he doesn't know how to eat?'" said Rudi, translating for his mother. After I finished, the family ate the leftover fish and rice, and I realized I had been eating everyone's meal.

When we prepared to return to school, Rudi's parents gave me a small knife as a present. It was all they had of value, and they wanted me to keep it to remember them. Rudi told me the visit was like a miracle for his family. They were so happy to have an American visit them. They kept touching my hair and my arms and laughing and staring until we got on the bus and waved to them. As I sat on the bus, I reflected on how I had made them happy just by visiting and sitting with them and sleeping on the floor with them. I realized how personal and unique are the events that bring happiness, but how universal are the shared emotions when you are in their presence, and how these emotions can ripple and engulf everyone around them. And something simple, like a small fish for dinner, can be the catalyst.

After I returned to the school, another student, Virginio, asked me if I'd like to visit his home, which was five hours by bus and then three hours by foot.

"Sure," I said.

We arrived dusty and tired after riding the bus and hiking over streams and along a rocky trail. Finally, at dusk we came to a clearing with five houses. As I enjoyed the pink and orange sunset, a woman suddenly appeared, spinning and dancing around me, circle after circle, around and around. She wore a brightly colored woven skirt, a simple white blouse, a jangle of beads around her neck, and large round metal earrings. Her face was dark with deeply etched lines, and her black hair hung in a long braid. She sang in high-pitched tones, with words I could not understand, and her eyes glowed with a profound happiness. She danced for fifteen minutes, and I stood transfixed, watching as the entire village now gathered around us. Round and round me she went, not allowing me to move.

After the woman stopped dancing, Virginio explained that when Americans liberated her village from the Japanese in 1945, she had made a pledge to God that she would dance around the next American to visit her village. Now, twenty-five years later, I was the next American. What she was feeling and doing when she had spun and danced around me had been stored up inside her for twenty-five years, and now I had released it. I was connected to those soldiers like an echo is connected to a voice miles away.

After a brief pause, the woman renewed her dance, and I noticed there were tears in her eyes and sweat on her face. And as she spun around me, I felt the moisture like tiny rain droplets.

Two years later, when they asked me at my Stanford medical school interview why I wanted to be a doctor, I did not remember the words of my grandfather or my mother. I remembered that woman.

I told my interviewer about the woman, the dance, and how it felt to be in the middle of the circle surrounded by sound and motion, to be connected to another time and other people who were no longer there, with a village of curious, smiling faces. I would never forget how the woman and the dance had swirled around me, almost lifting me off the ground that day.

"Isn't that what it's like to be a doctor?" I said. "To be in the center of the circle?"

He nodded. "Sometimes." He looked out the window wistfully.

Now my mind returned to the boys stabbed in the gang fight and a vision of them swirling around me. It was nothing like the woman who had danced, circling me in celebration.

I got up and walked into the bathroom. As I stood in front of the mirror over the sink, my face stared back at me, and I was shocked at how old and furrowed my face looked. My once-curly black hair had become gray, or at least mostly gray, and even the few dark patches had a clear destiny like the last few green leaves of a tree gone yellow in the fall. My long face now had lines, vertical around my mouth and horizontal on my forehead and at the corners of my eyes. My eyes still retained the strange multitoned colors of my youth. People who looked closely at my eyes would often remark, "Hey, you have two different-colored eyes. This one is green, and that one is brown." Actually, both my eyes had brown and green in them, but one had distinctly more green and the other, more brown. But they had often been the beginning of a conversation and an indication of how intently someone was looking at me. All of my former girlfriends had noticed it almost immediately. My body remained slim, no longer thin or skinny, as my mother would have described it in my youth, but still slim and fit from years of jogging after work. I had developed a bit of a stomach, but it could usually be hidden by the shirts I wore. If not for the gray hair, the lines on my face, and the stomach, it was essentially the same body I brought with me to Mexico when I was twenty-two years old.

I looked away from the image and opened a drawer to find a sleeping pill. I had a few Ambien left. They would do the job, and I'd wake up in eight or ten hours with my mind cleared of all the thoughts that were bouncing around inside now. It would be only a few minutes before I would begin to slip away effortlessly. I swallowed two pills and lay down again.

Now my mind moved to Mexico, where I had gone between finishing college and starting medical school. It was not a quiet, peaceful, floating sensation that I felt, but I didn't need that anymore. The pills would provide it.

Instead, I remembered the excitement and adventure of riding a horse across a swollen river, the knock at my window in the middle of the night summoning me to visit a place lit with lanterns and smelling of incense and herbs, and the experience of touching the body of a person to whom I was the only hope of escaping pain, suffering, or death. I became aware of the delicious sensations of fear, excitement, anticipation, and the unknown outcome like a scary movie. I could be the hero of my own adventures, secure that they would end in a deep, cleansing sleep no matter what dangers I might encounter along the way.

And then I heard the door opening and closing. It was my wife, back for her boxes. I pretended to be asleep, burying my head under the pillows. I knew it would be only minutes before I could not talk, when I would drift away.

"Dave, are you awake?" she asked.

"Yes," I mumbled.

"I just wanted to tell you I was here."

"Oh, thanks." I said.

"How was your night?" she asked.

"Terrible. There was a gang fight; two kids died."

"I don't know how you do it," she said.

"Neither do I," I said.

"But you like it," she said.

"I know. I think I must be sick. It's this strange sensation of excitement I get. I think it all started when I went to Mexico that very first time. It was like taking a test and figuring out an answer, and if I could do it, someone would live. But it's not true. I don't think I make much of a difference most of the time, and in the meantime, I have nothing left—for you, for the kids, for our life."

"That's not true. You're a wonderful dad. And you're a wonderful doctor. I . . . I just need my own space. It's not your fault."

"I don't know. Somehow I feel like I got on the wrong track. It's like I'm out there playing God, and who wants to be married to God? And it all started in Mexico. I still dream about it. Isn't that weird?"

"Well, I think you should go back there. And I've never thought I was married to God. A martyr perhaps, but not God. Maybe you'll figure it out." She collected her boxes. All of the important objects that symbolized our life together fit so easily into boxes, disappearing into the brown cardboard depths. The Jemez pot from our first trip together, the rocks, the photos, the shells from a vacation in Belize— all accumulated over years and so quickly gone. It was like packing up your desk at the end of the school year; what had been essential and central would soon become obscure and irrelevant. And the next year, you'd have new books and new friends—a new life.

"This is just stuff," she said. "It doesn't mean anything."

"Really," I said. "If it doesn't mean anything, why do you want it?"

My mind was fading, and I could barely keep my eyes open. I could feel the drug coming on, carrying me away. I wanted to say, "I want you," but the words would not come out. I wanted to tell her how each of those objects in the boxes represented my tenuous connection to her and our life together. I moved my lips, but there was no sound. I remember the look on her face, the faint smile.

"Sleep," she said. "Sleep."

Chapter Two

I SLEPT FOR EIGHT HOURS, AND WHEN I WOKE UP I TRIED TO remember what had happened before I went to sleep. Laura had been there, and we had talked about Mexico—about my going down to the village again—and as I was trying to remember what we said about it, the phone rang. It was Rick.

Usually, when the emergency department attending physician called me, it was for one of two reasons. Either something had happened in the department—a patient died whom we had sent home, a doctor or nurse was hurt by a patient—or the oncoming attending had not shown up at the appropriate time and could not be located. It was about the right time for that second type of call.

"The nurses told me about you, about your wife. I feel terrible. Why didn't you tell me?" Rick asked.

"I . . . I guess it's so personal, and I don't really believe it yet. I keep thinking she'll change her mind," I said.

"I don't want to pry, but if there's anything I could do . . . ?" he said.

"Well actually, I was thinking of going down to Mexico in a few weeks. I have a Friday and Saturday night shift I need to trade. You're working the Thursday night shift. Do you think you could do them?"

"Friday and Saturday night after a Thursday night? That's pretty tough. My wife told me I shouldn't do more than two nights in a row because I get so grouchy. But considering the situation, I'll do it."

"You will?"

"Sure."

"I'll make it up to you," I said.

"Oh, don't worry about it. But why do you want to go to Mexico? Why don't you just go out and buy her flowers?"

"Well, I need some space to think. And Mexico was the place I first got going on the doctor track. It was where I really decided to be a doctor. I'm wondering if there's some clue down there about why it turned out like this."

"Yeah, for me it was the army. Before that, I would have been a chemist or a physicist; but in Vietnam, with all the guys getting shot and bleeding, I changed my mind. But you still should get her flowers, take her out. That's what I did when my wife wanted to leave me."

"When did your wife want to leave you?" I asked.

"Lots of times."

"Really? I never knew," I said.

"No, I never told anyone," he said. "What about your kids? What did you tell them? What are you going to do with them?"

"I don't know," I said. "They cried. I mean their whole world is upside down. They wanted to know where they would sleep. Could they bring their clothes with them? Would we have to move?"

"That's terrible," he said. "We had our kids after years of trying. It was the best thing we've ever done. I always liked your wife. She was perky and a little wild. You were always too serious, but she had that wild streak, like a wild horse. When you two got married was the last time I wore my black suit. Do you have a girlfriend?"

"What? No, of course not."

"What about her?"

"Well, no; I don't think so."

"Maybe she'll come back."

"Maybe, but I'm not going to hold my breath," I said.

"You're not one to let go of something easily. I remember that study you did on sepsis where you had to review hundreds of charts. I told you it was impossible. But you did it, a few charts every week. I couldn't believe it. It must have taken a year."

"Two years, actually," I said and then continued. "I'm not letting go. Well, maybe I am. You know, sometimes you just have to accept reality. You can't have a marriage if only one person wants it. You need two. I mean, in the trauma room, I'll fight to save someone, particularly if it's a young person, as long as there's any chance. Maybe longer than that. But eventually you know. The eyes cloud over and the skin feels cold, and everyone begins to look at you, waiting for you to say it. To say, 'Stop.'"

"So you're ready to call the code," he said.

"I don't know. That's why I want to go to Mexico. To be able to take a step back, like in the trauma room, where you look at the monitors and the techs and nurses and blood and IV fluid, everything circling around the patient, who's lying on a stretcher in the middle of it all."

"Well, it's the best show in town. It's better than any of those shows on television. I mean, you couldn't make this stuff up. But we're getting too old for it. Just three years and I'll have my twenty-five years, and I can retire. I'll sort of miss all our drunks: Jimmy Anderson, Tommy Nieto, Mary Joe. They make me remember what could have happened to me. My dad used to drink, but my parents stayed together."

"Yeah, that's what people used to do. My parents got married after the war. They were from the same town. All their friends and family were from that town. They did what was expected of them: stay together, keep the family together unless it is really bad. Now, we trade each other in like cars every few years, for the newest model," I said.

"When maybe we only need to change the oil and wiper blades," he said.

Rick's last words continued to echo in the silence that followed. We had known each other for the past twenty years, handing off patients like the batons in a relay race. We were teammates, intimates, but we barely knew each other. He had never told me about his marriage. Finally he said, "You don't need to pay me back."

"For what?" I asked.

"For the shifts. For the Mexico shifts."

"Oh, thanks," I said.

"Well, I'll talk to you later."

"Bye."

"Bye."

As I wandered about my house, I began to page through the books and photo album that lay on the half-empty bookshelves. Laura and I had both wanted the photo album and ultimately agreed to share it, so that it would stay for a year at each house even though I had taken almost all the photos. There were my baby photos and my early school photos. And there was a photo of me in Mexico on a mule, wearing a cowboy hat, unshaven, with a macho grin on my face. I sat down, and it began to come back to me—how I got there and all the subsequent encounters with the people from the clinic, and the ways the experience carried through my life.

I had gone down to this clinic in the Sierra Madre of Mexico before starting medical school, to test my resolve about being a different kind of doctor—one who was not concerned about making money and who would use his skills to help those most in need, like the originator of the clinic, Carl Wilson. It was the time of the Vietnam War, after the assassinations of Martin Luther King and Robert Kennedy—a time of rejection of the military and the American flag. I read about the clinic in a newspaper article in 1972, during my last quarter at Stanford. I had just received my acceptance letter to Stanford medical school and was feeling a little hypocritical and guilty as my college friends joked with me about when I'd be buying my first Mercedes Benz and a house in Atherton.

"No, it's not like that," I'd say. "I'm not going to live like that."

"Yeah, right. That's what you said for your interview, but let's see where you are in twenty years."

When I read the article about Carl Wilson, I saw a living example of what I had been imagining. Carl Wilson, a medical missionary, had devoted the last three years of his life to building a clinic for poor Mexican farmers in the foothills of the Sierra Madre. Lacking electricity, clean water, and even the most basic medical care, the people had adopted the American clinic. The clinic operated on donations from Americans interested in helping the destitute villagers of this beautiful, isolated valley in the mountains.

"I provide basic medical care," said Wilson. "And the people take care of my needs. They built the clinic, and they provide food and housing for me and the other American volunteers who have assisted me. We do not charge for our services, but sometimes people will bring fruit from their trees, a chicken, or eggs, or they will help repair something at the clinic."

One comment in particular stuck in my mind. When asked why he had decided to devote his life to this village, Wilson had answered, "Well, maybe someday we will ask why all of us aren't doing this. We would sacrifice ourselves for others in a war. Well, this is also a war—against disease. It's really quite simple."

The article went on to describe a typical day at the clinic. Carl Wilson treated a baby dehydrated from diarrhea, a man with an infected wound from a machete, and a woman with pneumonia. All might have died without the clinic.

At the end of the article was an address where donations could be sent. I wrote a letter volunteering to help at the clinic and included a donation of twenty-five dollars to the foundation that supported it. A few weeks later, I received a handwritten letter from Carl Wilson.

Dear David,

Thank you for your donation of twenty-five dollars to La Clínica. Every penny donated will be used for vital medications and equipment for the villagers of the clinic. I understand that you are interested in volunteering to help at the clinic. Usually we are only able to accept fully trained physicians, but we recently lost one of our staff volunteers and could use some basic help if you are available now and for the next six months. Please contact us at the foundation office for directions to the clinic if you are available.

Fondly,
Carl Wilson

When I had written the brief note with my check, I had not imagined any response—and certainly not a positive one. Now I suddenly had to consider whether I was ready to leave the comfortable Stanford campus, my friends, and my graduation to travel to a rural village in Mexico where I would have to speak Spanish and help in a medical clinic even though I didn't have any actual medical skills. I would have to talk with my faculty advisors and my parents, move out of my dorm room, and figure out where I'd be living when I returned and whether I had enough money to live on while I was volunteering. It all seemed crazy and far too precipitous, but when I asked my advisor, my friends, and my parents, they all encouraged me to go. Even the medical school offered to allow me to attend an intensive suturing course and physical-diagnosis class with a group of physician's assistants over the next week. Several of my friends agreed to drive me to the clinic if I could get the directions.

"OK," I said to the woman who answered when I called the phone number written in my letter. "I'll go."

"Oh, good," she said. "Carl Wilson has always said that when the need is greatest, it pulls like a magnet. You were the one chosen."

She gave me directions about how to drive down the Pan American Highway, where to cross the border, which towns to pass (Hermosillo, Culiacán), the place where there would be a sign, and the long dirt road that would wind past farms and through arroyos before arriving at the village.

A week later two friends and I piled into a car loaded with sleeping bags, suitcases, donated medicines, stethoscopes, sodas, bananas, crackers, cheese, a Spanish dictionary, maps, toilet paper—all the necessities. We departed on a windy March morning, heading south.

"Let's spend a few nights on a beach," suggested Alan, one of my dorm mates. Although Alan was interested in medicine and curious about the clinic, he also wanted to enjoy the break from school. I also suspected that he was anticipating how uncomfortable his long, lanky body would feel after hours packed into the small car.

"I think they're waiting for me," I said.

"Look, man. I want to get my feet up and sip on a cold Tecate. I can almost taste it. There'll still be plenty of kids with diarrhea for you to put diapers on. There's supposed to be this beach near Hermosillo where fishermen bring you fresh fish, and girls walk around topless."

"I thought you were taking me down because you wanted to help the clinic," I said. "We've got this whole car full of donations. I'll buy you beer when we get across the border."

"What's wrong with combining business and pleasure?" asked Alan.

"We're supposed to be helping a guy who is like Albert Schweitzer. I don't think Albert Schweitzer was sitting on the beach."

We crossed the border at Mexicali and headed toward the Pan American Highway. The car began to smell of bananas and melting rubber from the food and stethoscopes roasting in the back window. We stopped to eat at a cantina with red checkerboard tablecloths covered with flies. I bought Tecates for Alan and my other friend, Nick, and we waited for our "Comida Mexicana" of frijoles, rice, and enchiladas.

"This place is fucking hot," said Alan as he sipped his Tecate. "I'd sure like to be on a beach now."

"Sorry, Alan," I said. "Just drop me off at the clinic, and then you guys can head for Mazatlán."

"Yeah, but we're passing beaches on the way. Beaches with topless girls from San Diego State."

"How do you know they're from San Diego State?" I asked.

"Because I know a girl from San Diego State, and she was the one who told me about the beaches where they all go," he said.

I looked at the nine-year-old wall calendar. The face of John F. Kennedy, former president of the United States, stared back at me. He stood guard over the year of 1963 as if his assassination could still be prevented. A painting of the Virgin Mary hung just above the wall calendar.

We paid for our meals in dollars and received pesos in change. I stared at the unfamiliar coins with faces of military heroes on one side and eagles and snakes on the other side. I realized how little I knew about Mexican history, the heroes of the revolutions, or even the president. My few words of Spanish—tortillas, cerveza, sombrero—had all crossed over into English usage.

We folded ourselves back into the car and resumed our ride. The road had slow-moving trucks, which we passed easily, and huge potholes. The smell of chicken and smoke from the roadside cooking stands mixed with the exhaust of buses idling by the side of the road and wafted through our windows. We passed the signs for *playas*—beaches—and Alan nodded to silently remind me of his sacrifice, or perhaps he was giving me another chance to change course. But I was now determined to reach the clinic in a state appropriate to the solemnity of the situation and my new role. I did not want to have to explain a side trip to a beach to people who were choosing to volunteer at a medical clinic.

We turned at the small, faded sign that pointed the way to the village. Immediately, the road deteriorated into a mélange of dirt and pavement, not exactly a dirt road, but one with so many ruptures in the asphalt that bumps were more common than smooth stretches. This was only a brief transition to a completely dirt road with deep gullies and with rocks jutting out through the dirt surface.

"Sorry, Alan," I said as we bounced from pothole to rock and over deeply rutted sand.

"You owe me big time," he said.

Clouds of dust washed over and through the car. Alan coughed, and then I coughed as I inhaled the dust and hurried to close the window.

But even with our air-conditioning, the car was too hot, and we gradually reopened the windows in spite of the dust clouds. Small adobe and stucco huts lined the roadway. Fences of cut tree limbs enclosed courtyards where chickens and barking dogs roamed. The fence posts, with clusters of leaves and branches growing out of the cut ends, created a living-fence shrub. A man on a horse trotted past us. He wore a yellow straw cowboy hat and a white cotton shirt. His face had the same shiny tan glow as his leather saddle. He stared at us through gray-blue eyes and then lifted his hand and waved. We all waved back.

"Hey, man, the next guy we'll see will probably be Zorro or the Lone Ranger," said Alan.

We saw no other cars on the road as we continued on past clusters of houses and the occasional cows or donkeys that wandered into our path. I wondered how the owners would track down their animals or whether they were like the sacred cows of India that could travel along roads without fear of anyone taking them. Finally, after three hours on the dirt road, we crested a hill covered with thorny, brown shrubs and low, flat cactus, and suddenly homes spread out before us. I could feel my pulse quicken as we entered the village. Houses crowded together on the main street, creating a colorful patchwork of pastel colors— turquoise, peach, gray, white, and pink. Pigs lounged along the edges of the road in pools of gray muddy water. Cobblestones replaced the dirt road surface as we entered the center of the village, and I heard the sharp clicking of horse hooves on the cobblestones as two men on horses trotted past. As I was about to suggest that we ask for directions to the clinic, I spotted a house with a sign: La Clínica. The sign was hand carved from a wooden slat and the letters were painted red. We parked the car and slowly unfolded and stretched our arms and legs. Several children gathered around the car, staring into the windows and touching the dusty surface. "Gringos, gringos!" they yelled out excitedly.

"Yup, the gringos are here," said Alan.

I unloaded my backpack and the boxes of donated medical equipment, bandages, stethoscopes, and ointments. I had also brought a sleeping bag, some peanut butter, and toilet paper.

After unloading the car, I stood outside the clinic with the gathering crowd of children and curious adults, several of whom looked like clinic patients.

"I think you better go in," said Alan. "I'll watch the stuff."

"OK," I said.

I passed through the waiting area, which consisted of a dark room with two long benches on either side and wall posters with instructions about breast-feeding, diarrhea, and vaccinations. The next room contained a central examining table, a desk, and two chairs. Shelves of medications were stacked along the walls with signs that identified them by diagnosis or symptom in English and Spanish: "Cough Medicine—*Tos*," "Stomachache—*Dolor del estómago*," and "Antibiotics—*Antibióticos*." Row after row, like books in a library. I was surprised to see a thick layer of dust covering the bottles of liquid and pills. An odor of disinfectant and mildew drifted up from the shelves.

In the middle of the room, gathered around the examining table, were four people. They appeared to be treating a baby with intravenous fluid that flowed from a bottle suspended from one of the wooden beams of the ceiling. As my eyes adjusted to the shadows and slits of light passing through the shutters on the windows, I realized that two of the people were probably the parents. The woman, no more than sixteen years old, wore a colorful embroidered blue and red skirt and a white cotton blouse. She had a hint of red in her brown cheeks, and her dark eyes looked down at the floor. The man with her seemed even younger, perhaps fifteen, with a white shirt, a red bandanna around his neck, and jet-black hair hanging down to his shoulders.

Next to them was Carl Wilson, the leader of La Clínica. Deep in concentration, he adjusted the intravenous fluid flowing into the arm of the baby, who lay on its back, wrapped in a green and red blanket. Carl Wilson wore jeans and a white T-shirt, and his bushy beard blended into tangles of long blond-brown hair. His posture seemed strained as he bent over the child, and when he straightened up to stare at the drip chamber in the plastic intravenous tubing, there was an awkward moment of imbalance. Next to him was a boy about twelve or thirteen, who appeared to be assisting—holding the child's arm still, or searching for tape or other supplies.

I stood silently watching for a minute before Carl Wilson turned around. As I met his gaze, I noticed his reaction of surprise and then displeasure.

"I'm David Sklar. I wrote to you, and you wrote me back and said you needed some help," I said.

"You're the student from Stanford?" he asked in a high nasal tone as his expression softened into an attempt at a brief smile before returning to a scowl. Stretching up on his toes like a huge bird, he scanned the room and noticed my two friends. Alan was bringing in boxes and examining the bottles along the wall.

"Oh," I said. "These are two of my friends who brought down some donations from Stanford medical school. There are stethoscopes, some bandages, and some burn ointment, I think."

"Did you bring any antibiotics?" he asked.

"No, I don't think so."

"We really need some antibiotics. This child needs antibiotics," he said, pointing at the child in the middle of the room.

"Oh," I said. "What's wrong with the baby?"

"We're not sure. It could be meningitis. Perhaps TB," he said. Then he took a few steps forward and extended his hand.

"Carl," he said as he grasped my hand. I was surprised at the tentative, probing nature of the handshake. His fingers felt thin and bony, and the middle of the palm lacked the usual fleshiness that made a handshake a squeeze. As he came close, I could smell the sweat and dust on his shirt.

"This is Luis," he said, pointing to the boy who had been assisting him. "Luis is from the village, but he speaks excellent English."

The boy approached me and extended his hand enthusiastically. He had dark brown hair and fair skin. His eyes sparkled with confidence and enthusiasm.

"I am very happy to meet you," he said. As he spoke, I realized he was probably closer to fourteen or fifteen than twelve. If not for his accent, I would have guessed he was from the United States. "I went to school in California for the eighth grade."

"Luis helps out here at the clinic. He's our local dentist," said Carl.

"Dentist?" I said. "I thought this was a medical clinic."

"Yes, well, disease does not distinguish whether a doctor, a dentist, or a physical therapist is needed. We do everything here. So what kinds of things can you do?"

"Well, I didn't have much time. I had a crash course on suturing, and I attended some classes for the physician's assistant course. But I'm really just starting medical school. Actually, I start in the fall. But I'll do whatever you need."

"Yes, well, we have books," he said and pointed to a set of text-books on the bookshelf between the bottles of medicines. I noticed an anatomy book, a book titled *Diagnosis and Treatment.* Another was called *Differential Diagnosis.* There were books on pediatrics, obstetrics and gynecology, surgery, and dermatology. "If you read the books and use common sense, you can figure most anything out. Anyway, let me take you around the clinic, and then you can take your things over to Ricardo and Rosa's house. They live right next to the clinic, and they have agreed to take you in. They are expecting you."

"OK," I said.

"Your friends . . . ," he said, pausing as he watched Alan opening bottles that sat on the shelf. "Your friends can go now, if they'd like. Luis can watch the baby while we walk around."

"Hey, Alan," I said. "You guys can head for the beach. I'll be OK. They're expecting me."

"Hey, cool," he said. "I mean, if you need us to stick around and do some surgery or something, we can. It's the strangest doctor's office I've ever seen. No one's even wearing a white coat. And it smells like a bus station."

"Yeh," I said. "It's pretty low-key. But I think you guys should shove off. Have a margarita for me."

"Hey, we'll have two or three."

"Thanks for driving all this way."

"No problem. Maybe you'll become some famous doctor, and I'll be able to say that I got you started down the right path and kept you from all those topless San Diego State girls on the playa."

"OK. Well, I think I need to start helping," I said as I turned toward where Carl was waiting for me.

"Be good," said Alan, and he hugged me as did Nick, my other friend. I heard the engine start as Carl began his tour of the clinic.

"The clinic has three rooms," he said. "There's the waiting room, which you passed through to get into this room. As we go back into the waiting room, you'll notice the benches. These benches fill up with patients early in the morning, and when they are full, that's how many patients we will see that day—except for emergencies, which we will see anytime. As you can see, all the benches are empty now because we had to send the last patients away when the baby arrived a few hours ago."

"I like the posters," I said.

"Yes, we are working with the local schoolteacher to encourage the students to draw good health posters, and we will display the best examples here at the clinic."

As Wilson explained about the posters and the school project, I had an opportunity to observe him. His eyes, recessed deep in his face, sparkled with energy as his hands gestured emphatically. His face was mostly a tangled beard with the blue eyes peering out. Deep furrows crossed his forehead when he raised his eyebrows as he talked. The bones of his face seemed to poke through thin skin, giving him a faintly skeletal appearance. He had placed a dirty yellow straw cowboy hat on his head, and the hat tipped precariously as if his hair were straining to free itself from the hat's constraints. His too-large T-shirt hung from his slender frame, and the metal part of a stethoscope encircled his neck, while the diaphragm extended down to his belt. His jeans were baggy, and he used a tight belt to keep them from falling down. His brown leather cowboy boots dug into the dirt as he walked.

As we entered the dental room, he pointed to the green dental chair. "This is where Luis works," he said and smiled. "An American dentist came down here for two weeks and taught him how to pull teeth. Now Luis teaches all of the volunteers how to pull teeth. He'll be teaching you."

"I'll be pulling teeth?" I asked.

"Oh, yes. In a day, you'll be able to do it. You'll be doing many things here."

"Where do all the supplies come from?"

"Oh, people bring them as donations, like you just did. Or we buy them with the money that people donate to the foundation." He showed me the dental supplies: cotton balls, sharp metal instruments, needles, and anesthetics. It could have been any dental office, if not for the dirt floor and dusty shelves.

"This is our laboratory," he said as he pointed to a corner of the dental room that had a microscope, a collection of bottles with colored liquids, and boxes of glass slides. "We can do gram stains, urinalyses, and blood counts. We even have a centrifuge, which we can use if we can get our generator going."

Next to the microscope were a laboratory manual and several books. Posted above the colored bottles were instructions on how to do a gram stain. Drawings of birds lay on the countertop, the subjects identified with captions: *Blue Heron in Rio Verde* and *Turkey Vulture Hovering over Chilar*. They were exquisite in detail and delicate. "Who did these?" I asked.

"Oh, I doodle a bit," he said.

"They're beautiful," I said, and then I noticed a drawing of two hands, the bones and veins like hills and rivers of a peninsula. The hands appeared to be reaching out to touch something, but they were frozen in space, disembodied. They brought to mind the stories of how thieves in Saudi Arabia, Iraq, Iran, and Syria had their hands amputated as punishment for their crimes. The hands were beautiful, eerie, and disturbing. They were his hands. I wondered why we have pictures of people's faces, but almost never pictures of hands or feet.

We walked out into a courtyard enclosed by a covered portal. "Families stay here when a patient needs to spend the night. We have cots, and we set them up here in the portal. The families help provide the nursing care. We have a little generator in the back corner for when we need electricity for the centrifuge or the X-ray machine."

"You have an X-ray machine?" I asked.

"Yes, we are quite well-equipped. However, we have run out of film. Above us is a loft where I have some clothes and a few cots for when I need to sleep here at the clinic. Usually I spend the night at someone's home, and the volunteers are usually invited to stay at a local family's home too. But occasionally we use the loft."

When we returned to the room with the baby, I noticed another man, with a white moustache and short gray hair. "*Oiga, oiga*," he said. Listen, listen.

"*Pásale*," said Carl. Come in.

The man described how his wife had suddenly begun to mumble. He could not understand her speech. And she could not walk; she just sat in a chair mumbling. I could understand about half the Spanish and could understand Carl's questions better than the man's answers.

"I need to go with this man to see his wife. I would like to take Luis with me in case I need any help. Do you mind staying here with the baby?"

"What do I have to do?"

"Just make sure the IV solution continues to drip. The baby is dehydrated and needs the fluid, but there should not be much for you to do. We should be back soon," he said.

"Sure, no problem," I said with a forced bravado.

I watched as they gathered up medical equipment and medications and put them into a woven bag with a strap. Luis carried the bag.

"This is how you make the drops go," said Luis as he showed me how to adjust the flow rate. "As long as the little drops keep going, it's OK. If the drops stop, then maybe you have to move the hand where the needle is. But you move it just a little, so the needle will not go out of the vein." He showed me how to move the child's hand gently.

As I got close to the baby and the parents, I noticed the smell of sweat and dirt and horsehair and breast milk.

Luis wore a T-shirt and jeans, and with his shoulder-length brown hair, he could have been a teenager at any high school in the United States. He slouched a bit as he walked and liked to flash a toothy smile as he talked.

"Come on, Luis," said Carl. "We're taking the Jeep."

Luis pulled a key from his pocket. "This is the key to the Jeep," he said proudly.

I watched as Carl and Luis left the clinic, and I heard the motor start and the Jeep roll down the street. As the noise of the engine faded, I realized there were no other vehicles driving on the street, no other engines. There was also no electricity anywhere, no lighting for the clinic. I realized the room would soon be dark. I looked at the parents, standing silent vigil next to me. The man's face, dark and glistening, mostly in the shadow of his black hat, stared at the woman in her long dress and then at the baby and at me.

"Light?" I said hopefully in Spanish.

They smiled. They were so young, too young for a baby, particularly a sick baby. And too trusting, to leave their baby under my care.

"*¿Luz?*" I repeated. Light?

They smiled again, smiles of innocence and ignorance, and I smiled back.

We stood in the gathering darkness, watching the clear intravenous fluid drop into the plastic tubing connected to the baby's hand. Drop, drop, drop, drop. I had no idea what the purpose of the fluid might be, but I began to believe in the importance and inevitability of each drop, like the ticks of a clock. Each drop meant I was closer to the time when Carl would return.

Then the baby began to shake. It shook as if possessed by an evil, nonhuman force that wrenched and squeezed its tiny body. I watched in terror. Everything was happening so fast. The parents rushed up to the baby, and the father made the sign of the cross as the mother began to cry. She was just a child herself. In the darkness the baby's eyes glowed a soft white, and I thought, "This must be what death looks like." I touched the baby's head to keep it from banging. Then it was quiet. I thought the baby was dead. But then the eyes returned to normal, and suddenly the baby began to breathe again, deep noisy breaths, but at least they were breaths. The parents looked at me as if I had stopped the seizure. The hand I had placed on the baby's head had accomplished a miracle.

"Gracias," the father said, and his eyes swept from me to the ceiling in search of a divine presence.

I noticed that my hands were shaking.

It was now fully dark. I could no longer see the drops from the IV. I could only stand staring at the baby, waiting to see what might happen next. The lights of the returning Jeep created eerie shadows as it slowed and parked in front of the clinic. Carl and Luis came into the clinic with flashlights.

"What happened?" Carl asked, noting that the child's condition had changed and that we were standing around anxiously. Before I could answer, he said, "Luis, get the lantern."

"I think the baby had a seizure," I said. "It started shaking; its arms, its legs, and its head were banging against the table. I touched the head, and the shaking stopped."

"The IV came out," he said. "We'll have to start another."

"I'm sorry. I didn't notice," I said.

Carl probed the tiny vein in the dim lantern glow and inserted a catheter, a long thin piece of plastic that slid over a needle. His fingers trembled slightly as he gathered up the plastic-and-paper envelope that had kept the catheter sterile. The drops began to flow again, and we taped the tubing securely to the wrist and put a cardboard splint on the hand to keep it from bending or moving.

"What was wrong with the woman?" I said.

"What woman?" he said absently.

"That woman who was mumbling, who could not speak or move."

"Oh, she is diabetic. She took too much medicine. We gave her some juice and she came out of it, and then she wanted to serve us all dinner, so we had to eat a few cookies with her," he said.

"Oh, that's good," I said.

"So you want to go to medical school," he said.

"Yes, I think so."

"Waste of time, medical school. They never teach you about cases like this in medical school."

"Why?" I asked.

"Because medical school is about hospitals, money, and power. But this is where most of the people in the world live. This is where they come for care—poor rural outposts in clinics like ours. Who is going to teach you about them? Medical school is about hoarding knowledge, making people pay, scaring them into thinking they will die if they don't pay. And it's about convincing people that you have to be some kind of genius to be a doctor. Anyone can be a doctor. Just come to a place like this, get some books, and start helping people. That's what it's all about."

"But how can you help people if you don't know what you're doing?" I said, remembering how helpless I felt when the baby was shaking.

"Look, doctors take credit every time the patient gets well, even if they didn't know what was wrong or how the condition got better, like the seizure that stopped by itself," he said. "And they make people pay and pay. Even poor people who have nothing. Here we just help them. We care about them, and they care about us. They bring food. They built the clinic. It's love that makes this place work. They don't teach that in medical school. They never will."

I stood watching the IV, unable to reply. I wondered if I had made a mistake about medical school. I had imagined that I could help people and still make a living, and I expected to treat people even if they could not pay. But Carl was implying that any active involvement in the medical system was unacceptable. "But why should anyone do it, work in a place like this for nothing?"

"Doctors will not do it," he said. "Doctors are not the answer. Certainly they can help. There will be people who are committed, or others who may volunteer for a time because they want to blot out their guilt for getting rich on people's misery, but doctors are not the answer. Medical school is not the answer."

"What is the answer?"

"We need to re-create the whole world, village by village, community by community, and country by country. The medical clinic is only one piece of what we need to do."

I stood in the lantern light watching the shadows flickering. I did not understand what he was talking about, and I felt the lateness of the night and the long trip.

Finally, Wilson said, "I'm going to lie down for a while in the loft in back. Luis can stay here with you," and he disappeared through a door. He did not wait for me to respond or agree.

Luis came over to me. He bounced slightly when he walked, as if he were walking on a cushion. He stood next to me and smiled as if we were friends. I smiled back awkwardly because I did not feel happy.

"Very serious," he said.

"The baby?" I said.

"Yes, and Carlos also," he said, referring to Carl Wilson.

"Carlos," I said. "Carlos. You call him Carlos?"

"Sure," he said.

"How do you know Carl?" I asked.

"I met him when he came here three years ago. Now he's like my father."

"Oh," I said. "Does he have any family, any children, or a wife?"

"No. He has a brother. But we are his family," he said.

I had heard of doctors who had devoted themselves to a town, who lived there for their entire lives and never married. It seemed like a lonely life, but it also reminded me of the lives of monks, priests, and other religious devotees who abandoned earthly pleasures in exchange for spiritual fulfillment. "I've never been to a place like this," I said. "It's such a different world."

"Yes, it's not beautiful like California," he said.

"No."

"It's Mexico."

"What do you think about the baby?" I asked.

"I think the baby is OK now."

"Yes, I hope so," I said.

"Well, I'm going to take my rest now. Then I will come back," he said.

As I waved goodnight to him, I watched our shadows in the flickering lantern light and stared at the line of intravenous tubing, an uncertain, insubstantial connection to the baby's bottle of fluid: drop, drop, drop, drop. You could barely see the drops in the shadow, each one helping to sustain the baby through the night. My mind ranged over many landscapes as I sat there trying to make sense of the night, giving up, finally, as I blinked my eyes.

Every time I closed my eyes and opened them again, I was surprised to find myself there with the baby, with the parents lying on a blanket in the corner, snoring. Carl and Luis were sleeping in the back. I felt like I was trespassing in another world. It was different from going away to Stanford or the Philippines because even though they were different worlds, there I had not been responsible for anyone but myself. I wondered if this was what being a doctor felt like: to be alone for a moment with a fragile life, as if it were mine for a moment. I stayed awake the rest of the night amid a symphony of thoughts that would reverberate every night that I was awake with sick patients. I thought about my fatigue, my uncertainty, my endurance, the sound of my breathing, the unsteadiness of my hand, and about not giving in to sleep. I thought about the baby, his chest and stomach moving up and down with each breath, the disease inside his body. I thought about the linkage between us, tenuous and random and melting away like a dream. Ever since that night, I have been pursuing moments like that—when my life suddenly seemed to become larger, its purpose connected to the life of another. Ever since that night, I have been chasing a phantasm that appears and disappears, grotesque or beautiful depending upon the light and shadows.

That night the parents, the baby, Carl, and Luis all slept. Only I was awake to hear the roosters and watch the clinic emerge in the early morning light.

Chapter Three

THE RECOLLECTION OF THAT FIRST DAY AND NIGHT RELEASED many fragmentary memories: the sounds of hands slapping tortillas and the smell of the tortillas roasting over an open fire; the feel of a horse between my legs, running full out; a face of death staring up at me.

I sat in a daze and let the images continue rather than think about the meetings and problems I would have to address at work the next day. I had slept all day and was not ready to go back and sleep more. My head was still a little cloudy, but I remembered what had happened at the clinic the second day. It all came back: the next day, the next week, and beyond.

My second day at the clinic began with the appearance of a man with one arm, who entered the clinic and started to sweep the floor. "*Buenos días,*" he said, laughing as he moved his broom back and forth in front of me.

"Buenos días," I answered tentatively, standing protectively in front of the baby.

"It's just Loli," said Carl, who had walked up behind me. "Loli lost his arm in an accident. He helps out here at the clinic, like several of our former patients. He's harmless."

"Loli no speak English," said Loli. "Only sing a song. I be working on the railroad. All de liblog day. You like my song?" He smiled, showing a mouth with three scattered teeth.

I smiled back.

Carl examined the baby for a few minutes and then nodded to me.

"OK, let me find a place for you to sleep. I think Ricardo and Rosa are expecting you. The baby is better, so we all need to rest." Carl's eyes were bloodshot, and he was in the same clothes he had worn during the night.

We walked over to the house next door. A blue-eyed man with a three-day growth of beard shook my hand. His head looked small, perched upon broad shoulders and a deep chest. "Ricardo Montes, *a sus órdenes*," he said solemnly, as if presenting himself for duty to a commanding officer. "*Pase*." He motioned me into his house. He walked with his legs bowed out, as if he had been riding for days. His heels clanged with silver spurs. His wife, Rosa, grinned at me as she extended her hand in welcome. My hand was still throbbing from her husband's handshake when I squeezed her hand. Rosa had a soft, pear-shaped body loosely covered by a tan dress. Long black hair pulled back and twisted into a braid topped her round, dimple-cheeked face. Her clear, deep brown eyes examined me as if I were a new piece of furniture shipped from a great distance. She and Carl conferred in rapid Spanish before she led me into a room with a cot against the wall. A window with wooden shutters and metal bars opened out into an alley that adjoined the clinic.

"*Muchas gracias*," I said and moved toward the cot—made up with a sheet and a light cotton blanket—before I could notice my hunger. I was asleep in minutes in spite of the noises of horses trotting and people talking in the street. It was a jagged sleep. I would wake up, feel hungry, have no idea where I was, and then fall back asleep. Hours later, as the daylight was fading, Rosa knocked at the door and motioned me to follow her. She walked with a gliding, shuffling gait across the dirt floor. I followed her into a dim, lantern-lit room furnished with a table and chairs. This was the kitchen and dining room. Rosa began smacking and patting at dough in a stone bowl and placed it on a flat surface over a smoky wood fire. I gulped down watery beans with steaming tortillas. The tortillas had a grainy, rich taste almost like hot whole wheat pancakes. There were no utensils. I used the tortillas as rudimentary spoons and dripped bean juice on the table. No one else was eating with me, though I knew Rosa and Ricardo had six children. Later I learned that it was their custom to eat in shifts. Usually, I would be invited to eat with Ricardo. But for this first dinner, I was alone, too tired and disoriented to ask questions. I just ate and returned to my room where I resumed my bizarre dreams. When

I woke up, I heard roosters crowing and the scratching of brooms on the street.

Rosa had breakfast waiting for me—eggs and tortillas with refried beans. Her oldest son, eleven-year-old Tomás, sat at the table with me, smiling shyly as I attempted to practice my Spanish on him.

"*¿Escuela?*" I asked. School?

He nodded. That would be the extent of the conversations I would have with many people during that first week.

Rosa would pepper me with questions, and I would understand only a few words. I learned a way to parry questions without appearing stupid. I had heard certain expressions that seemed to appear in almost every conversation, and I began to use two phrases to maintain a conversation without admitting my ignorance. Anyone hearing me would assume I had understood whatever was being discussed.

"*¿Quién sabe?*" I'd say sometimes. Who knows? And other times I'd say, "*Como no.*" Of course. The expressions seemed to convey familiarity and only rarely got me into trouble.

That morning, Rosa asked whether I had slept well.

"Como no," I said.

Then she asked if I liked frijoles and eggs mixed together.

"¿Quién sabe?" I answered.

She nodded and proceeded to mix the eggs and beans.

She asked me my religion.

"¿Quién sabe?" I said.

"Are you Catholic?" she asked.

"Como no," I said.

She nodded, satisfied.

I thanked her for breakfast and went out to the clinic.

Weeks later, when I tried to explain to her that I was Jewish, she reminded me of this conversation and concluded that I was both Catholic and Jewish.

As I entered the clinic, Gabriel, a young man of about twenty, greeted me. He had the cracking voice of an adolescent or an old man, and his physical features had elements of both youth and age.

He walked stiffly, with a crutch in one arm, and extended an arthritic hand to me.

"Buenos días," he said. Gabriel assisted at the clinic, helping to write and file medical records for clinic patients. He had lived in a shuttered, unlit room, incapacitated by his swollen, painful joints and abandoned by his parents. Carl had learned about him and offered him steroid medication, which acted like oil on rusted metal, allowing his elbows, hips, knees, and fingers to bend for the first time in years. However, his face and torso became rounded from the medication while his arms and legs remained thin, giving him the appearance of a snowman. I asked him about the bathroom. I tried several words before he nodded and pointed me to the alley between the clinic and Ricardo and Rosa's home.

"At the end of the road," he explained slowly to me.

I wondered what I would find.

At the end of the road was a cliff, which overlooked the river a hundred feet below. Across the river, mountains rose up in the distance, and I would have enjoyed the view if not for the strong odor of human waste. Pigs roamed among the saplings that marked the end of the road. I looked in both directions and saw no outhouse. A young man passed me carrying a stick, almost a club. I watched as he took down his pants, squatted, and relieved himself. As he walked back past me, he handed me his club.

"For the pigs," he said.

I stood at a decision point; the odor of feces and urine was unmistakable as the pigs cleaned the cliff of its human waste.

Sitting all night with a baby, speaking Spanish, sleeping on a canvas cot, eating without a fork or spoon—all had seemed possible. But the indignity of squatting in the open while fighting off pigs and exposing myself to whoever walked along just seemed out of the question. With my stomach grumbling and my bladder bursting, however, I realized there was no other choice. I dropped my pants to my ankles and squatted down, holding on to a sapling.

A huge pink and black pig came running toward me, and I swatted at it, trying to finish as quickly as possible. The pig barely noticed my blow, and I swung again, harder. Falling back, I imagined myself plunging over the cliff with my pants down, my corpse discovered amid the rocks and toilet paper.

An old woman with white hair appeared from nowhere. "*Pégale*," she said. Hit him. And she swatted the pig away from me. This was doña Mercedes, who sometimes visited the clinic for entertainment.

She would put a chair next to the window so that she could observe dental extractions. Today, I was the entertainment.

"Gracias," I said.

Back at the clinic, Carl had decided that we should build a latrine. I could immediately see the value in the project. He distributed picks and shovels to the family of the baby with the seizures, my patient from the first night. The family members cheerfully dug down into the hard-packed clay soil, and now I became aware of a physical strength that had not been perceptible that night in the clinic. They introduced themselves to me: the baby's father, uncle, and grandfather. Each one descended into the enlarging hole, muscles glistening with sweat as they dug. They thanked me for curing the baby that night. Ricardo appeared and decided to pitch in, tearing into the hard soil with the pick as if trying to kill it. Drops of sweat covered his arms and chest. I tried to help, but my soft hands became red and blistered quickly. Ricardo's hands were rough with calluses.

When Carl appeared, we were resting, exhausted. He grabbed a pick and jumped into the hole, attacking furiously. Only a few minutes at his flailing pace would have gained respect and praise, but he continued until all of us were embarrassed and guilty about resting. When he finally emerged, dirty and sweating, he plunged the pick into the ground as a challenge. This was his way—to lead by example, to demonstrate what was possible. They all talked about him and gave him a title of respect—don Carlos—as if he had magical powers. Patients would tell me he could see through a body and heal with his fingers. He could make a tumor shrink away. He could make an old man young. And it was not only the villagers who set him on an altar; we all did. I know I did.

A musician named Gerónimo sat down next to the hole and began playing his guitar to provide a rhythm for the shovelers who now took up Carl's challenge. Gerónimo's bushy black eyebrows joined at his broad nose. As he hooted and sang, an echoing cry could be heard from the deepening hole. Luis came over to me. "He has diabetes. He sings best when his sugar is high. So he doesn't like to take his insulin."

"Oh, como no," I said, grateful for the information but confused by it.

A tall pediatrician from California named Dr. Silva arrived, accompanied by Tony, a balding young man holding a movie camera. Dr. Silva was assisting in the clinic for a few weeks and had been away visiting other outposts in the mountains. He explained that at some villages eight or ten hours away by mule, he was the first pediatrician ever to have visited. He discovered strange cases and saw syndromes that he had only read about in textbooks. He loved the rides on the mountain trails, the surprise of each new village, and the amazement in people's eyes when he would arrive with his stethoscope and bag of medicines. Numerous doctors from the United States would visit the clinic for a few weeks of adventure and then leave, but Dr. Silva had already made several visits.

Tony, a filmmaker from California, jumped around filming Gerónimo from different angles. His aim was to make a movie that could help with fund-raising. He winked at me as he filmed the latrine. "This is great. It's so real." He moved nervously, erratically, as he shifted his camera. He had dark, narrow eyes and thin brown hair, which he would cover with his hand intermittently.

"Yes," I said. "You'd never see so much enthusiasm about a latrine back home."

"Exactly. The spirit. It's Carl Wilson, of course, but it's also the people here."

"Yes," I agreed. "There are so many people here from all over. I had no idea. How did you end up here?"

"Oh, I've known Carl a long time. He's been like a big brother to me. He invited me to visit and shoot some film, fix broken equipment, and help out."

"Well, I can't dig anymore. My hands . . ." I showed him my blisters—shreds of skin and red ovals on my fingers.

"Don't sweat it," he said. "It's time for a siesta." He laughed as he walked away filming the músico, the hole, and all of us sitting around. I worried that the blisters on my hand were merely the most obvious manifestation of my softness, my unfitness to work here with the others. Everyone else seemed to have a purpose, but I felt useless. One night I was confused and alone with a sick baby, and the next, I was unable to dig a latrine. For a while I worried about it and then felt a lethargy from the sun's warmth and the rhythmic beat of shoveling. Relieved to see the latrine materializing before my eyes, I drifted into the song of the músico and the beat of digging down deep into the earth.

Chapter Four

THE VILLAGE WAS PERCHED ON A LOW BLUFF OVERLOOKING a river that drained part of the nearby Sierra Madre. Tiny hamlets of three or four adobe houses dotted the horse trails that led up out of the village, but the village itself was the end of the road. Large lorries lumbered through the unpaved streets before unloading their goods, which were sold at family tiendas, each tienda usually no more than a counter attached to a house. Sometimes trucks would arrive at night, unload, reload, and leave before the first light. Some people said it was related to drugs or some other illegal activity, but the business transacted was never discussed or apparent the next day at the tiendas. Most family members, including children, took turns at the tienda selling sodas, candy, rope, tools, soap—essentials and luxury items— to the village residents and the village's frequent visitors. These visitors would often ride for hours to fill saddlebags with canned fish, bread, or powdered milk. I wondered what they traded in return: perhaps a bag of grain. Larger goods were packed onto the backs of mules for transport up into the mountains. Tables, chairs, beds, and boxes full of food might be seen protruding from the backs of mules, attached with twine or leather strapping. Ricardo specialized in difficult pack-mule trips when he wasn't busy overseeing his herd of cattle. On this, my first weekend in the village, he invited me along for a short pack trip. He told me that he had already discussed it with don Carlos and received permission for me to go.

Noticing my hesitation, he said, "Don't worry. I'll give you the gentle female. Just hit her with the stick if she won't go."

I wasn't used to hitting animals with sticks, neither mules nor pigs.

I nodded, afraid to admit to him that I had never ridden a horse or mule. He hoisted me onto the saddle, and I clutched at the saddle horn as the mule took two steps forward. Ricardo handed me the reins and began to laugh.

"You don't have to hold her like your wife," he said.

As we proceeded forward, the slow sideways movements of the saddle developed a pattern that I could recognize. But the bump, bump, bump of a trot always seemed to bounce me around so that I received maximal impact. Two men on mules appeared suddenly from the bush and greeted Ricardo with a whistle and salutation.

"*Bienvenido, amigo.*" They welcomed him.

"This is my friend, David," he said, "who is living in my house. He is a doctor."

I bowed my head and removed my cowboy hat.

"*Mucho gusto*," they both said.

"David, I have some business with these men," said Ricardo. "*Momentito.*" Back in a moment. And he rode off, leaving me with the mules. A few minutes later, he returned and we continued up the trail. "Those were muchachos from Chilar," he said. "I have many friends in Chilar. They wanted some beer." The cargo we carried, covered in burlap bags, caused the mules to groan as they swayed and picked their way over sharp rocks along the narrow trail. The cargo was beer for a party, which was usually prohibited except for a fiesta day, which this happened to be. There would be parties up and down the mountain trail and a big celebration back at our village. Connections between people traveling the isolated mountain trails were as likely as connections between people who took the same train to work every day, though they were not so apparent to me.

"It's the fiesta of San José. We can drink beer and dance all night," Ricardo said.

I hadn't thought about dancing since I arrived at the clinic. It didn't seem right to think about dancing when there were people sick and in pain all around me.

But as we delivered our cargo at a small store, I began to think about it. What kind of music would there be? Rock and roll? Traditional Mexican music? I had always felt self-conscious at dances. Who would dance with me? Would everyone be watching? And then I realized

I'd hardly seen any girls in the town. Were there any? As the mule swayed and bounced, Ricardo began to sing about how much he liked to dance, how much he liked music.

When we arrived back at the village, a band of five men with guitars, horns, and an accordion were setting up to play on the plaza. Ribbons of red and white paper encircled trees and benches. Two outdoor restaurants appeared, offering cases of beer, tacos, and frijoles for sale. Clusters of men laughing and drinking beer paraded around girls in long white dresses with red and black sashes. I was amazed at the number of young girls, who smiled as they chatted with each other. Where had they been hiding?

I asked Ricardo why drinking was prohibited except for fiesta days.

"We've had some problems. When we drink beer, someone gets hurt. Two years ago a boy got shot because he was dancing with another boy's girlfriend, and since then, they have prohibited beer."

Tony and Luis arrived, and we watched as the men continued to empty can after can of beer, tossing the empty cans out into the road or crushing them on the ground.

Finally the music began to the wild hoots of delight from the men, who moved quickly to select dancing partners. All around the plaza, couples danced ranchero style to the jerky beat. Ricardo and Rosa danced up to me, glowing and twirling.

"How I love the music!" Ricardo said. Then he pointed to a dark, heavyset woman standing with two young children. "David, that woman, Chona, likes you. Go dance with her."

I nodded and smiled in Chona's direction out of courtesy. Then Tony walked over and took Chona for a spin around the plaza.

"Thanks," I said to Tony for standing in for me. "I don't know how to dance like this."

"Well, you better learn fast, because I'm getting my camera to do some filming, and you're going to represent us gringos." Tony arched his eyebrows high up on his forehead to emphasize his point, and I began to worry about yet another skill I lacked.

Deanna, a young woman who helped at the clinic, approached me. She smiled, revealing two gold front teeth, and dimples in her round cheeks. "I'll teach you," she said. But before I could answer, Tony grabbed her hands and began spinning her around in some kind of fancy dance step. "What a dancer, Antonio," she said, gasping.

I bought a beer for Luis and myself after he convinced me that he had been drinking beer since he was thirteen, and it was no big deal. The beer tasted particularly good in the oppressive heat, and I felt my sore muscles relaxing as I swallowed. Deanna returned, ready to teach me to dance, and we began bouncing and spinning. I felt the sweat on her neck and back as I held her, and I realized I had barely touched any women since I had arrived. The effect was immediate and overwhelming. Just as I began to enjoy dancing, I stepped on her feet for the third time, and she lost her enthusiasm and decided to teach me by having me watch her dance with Luis. Tony appeared with his camera and began filming.

At that moment a fight broke out. At first I thought it was an out-of-control dancing couple who had careened into others. But then two men tumbled to the ground, smashing beer cans on each other's heads. Family members and friends joined in, and the entire dance divided into warring parties, except for the young girls, who scampered home. Two of them, with dark eyes and long hair, stopped to stare at me. Deanna grabbed my hand.

"Let's go back," she said as I stared at the girls, who now, abandoned by their partners, seemed lost and adrift.

She pulled me as I looked back over my shoulder at the spectacle. When we finally arrived back at the clinic's doorway, Deanna disappeared to find a lantern. I stood against the door as a dark figure stumbled toward me and collapsed in a heap. One of the original combatants, he now lay bleeding from his head. Deanna helped me drag him into the clinic and put him on the examining table. All I could see was blood covering his eye, forehead, and nose. And then I began to feel dizzy, and I crumpled to the floor.

Dr. Silva—the visiting pediatrician—and Carl were there when I woke up. "Time for you to show us how you stitch," said Dr. Silva.

"I don't know. I feel kind of dizzy," I said.

"Well, there are two of them that need stitching, and more to come. So we need your help."

I got up slowly as my eyes tried to focus. The boy's wound had been washed and cleaned, and with the blood gone, it didn't look so bad. Just a cut above the eyebrow. The patient looked about my age, with bloodshot eyes, and so drunk that he did not move as I anesthetized the wound and placed five nylon stitches. I sutured in a daze, driving the needle through the skin, tying the knot, cutting, again and again. I hardly realized what I was doing, that this was a real person, until I was finished, or I might have hesitated and stopped. Dr. Silva checked my work and nodded approval. By the time I finished, the dance was over. All the girls were gone. The musicians were walking through the village, with their instruments mostly packed. And I had just finished cleaning mine. The needle holder, the scissors, the pickups all lay in antiseptic solution, soaking. I admired their precision and beauty as I absorbed the immensity of what I had just done, as if I had been using a magical power for the first time. This was my first surgical procedure, the first time I had sewn. I felt like singing or dancing to celebrate this event, but it was too late, too quiet. So I assumed a somber, serious expression befitting a doctor. I imagined that if I looked a certain way, I would become that way.

"Very nice," said Deanna, complimenting me as she left to return to her house. I nodded and thought of her hand in mine, the lingering touch.

There was a strange silence on the road punctuated by an occasional solitary burst of sound from a horn or guitar and then silence again. Ricardo came up to offer me a can of beer. When I declined, he opened it and drank it down. "I love the music," he said. "I really love the music."

And he danced off down the street, turning in circles as he went, saying over and over, "How I love the music."

Chapter Five

WHEN YOU SLEEP ALL DAY, YOU WAKE UP IN THE EVENING hungry and confused about what time it is and where you are. That's how I felt as I found myself in Albuquerque rather than Mexico, where my thoughts had been.

I got up from my seat, put the photo album down on the floor, and shuffled over to the refrigerator. I pulled it open and stared in at moldy cheese, salad dressing, eggs lining the door, cans of dark German beer, and containers of orange juice and milk. I grabbed two eggs and decided to make breakfast because I had just woken up even though it was night. I fried them up, grabbed a beer, and sat back down with the photo album. I paged through the pictures of the kids: Ethan and Ariel as babies and Laura as a young mother, when her hair was long. I remembered all those long nights when the children were babies, getting up at night with bottles. Laura wouldn't hear them, but I would. So I'd get up and sit with them and come back to her. She'd still be sleeping and would roll over to me in the bed and mumble something and fall back asleep.

I paged back past those pictures to the pictures of Mexico. There were faces of volunteers who showed up for a few days and then never returned. But they were there in the album, and they had their own stories. There was a picture that caught my eye of two girls in front of a van—Katherine and Linda. I could almost hear the excited screams of children the day they arrived: "*¡Gringitas!*"

I had been in the clinic with Carl, and Loli ran in shouting, "Gringitas, gringitas!" and swinging his one arm wildly. I followed him outside in time to see two girls emerge from a flowered VW van, stretching, yawning, and combing their hair. A crowd of men and boys gathered quickly around them and stared silently. The girls towered over the villagers. One of the girls, almost six feet tall, with long straight blond hair, addressed the crowd in English. "I'm looking for Dr. Wilson. He works in the *clínica*."

"Hi," I said. "My name is David. I work with Carl Wilson."

"I'm Katherine," said the tall girl extending her hand forward to shake mine. "And this is Linda."

"I'm Luis, and you are very welcome to come to my village," said Luis, who had suddenly appeared.

As the press of the curious villagers closed in around us, I said, "Come into the clinic with me," and led them through the door.

Carl stood up slowly to greet them.

Linda came forward and looked at the shelves of medicines. "Is this the clinic?" she asked.

"Yes, this is the clinic," Carl answered.

"OK. Well, we have some boxes of medicines from my dad for the clinic. They're out in the van."

"Oh, thank you," said Carl.

"I'm Linda Guffy; my dad is Dr. Guffy."

"Oh, yes. Dr. Guffy, from San Mateo."

"Portola Valley."

"Oh, yes. You are the high school girls from Portola Valley."

Linda grimaced and looked at her friend. Linda had a deeply tanned round face with black eyeliner accentuating her large brown almond-shaped eyes. When she grimaced, her pale lips lifted up to reveal teeth with metal braces. "Is there any water here?" she said. "I'm really thirsty."

"Well, we have water, but since you'll only be here a short time, you might as well avoid the water and drink sodas. The store down the road has Cokes, Fantas, and Sprite," said Carl.

Luis jumped forward. "Come with me. I'll show you."

As they departed, Carl began to shake his head. "I never thought they'd come. Their parents donated money to the clinic and mentioned something about donating antibiotics, but I never told them to send these girls. I wonder how they found us. We have no place for them. I can't be responsible for them." He talked to me as if I were a hotel concierge whom he wanted to remove an unpleasant guest, because he couldn't face the task himself.

The girls returned with boxes of antibiotics. Carl opened them and called out, "Tetracycline, ampicillin, erythromycin," as he examined individual bottles. "Very nice."

As he began placing the newly arrived antibiotics on the clinic shelves, he turned suddenly and announced, "I need to leave the clinic for a few hours. David will be in charge while I'm gone. If I'm not back by nightfall, please make yourselves comfortable in the clinic. And thank you for all of these wonderful medicines." He then put a few more bottles on shelves before assigning the task to the girls and me.

Katherine asked me how she could help. I had her sort antibiotics into groupings, for easier shelving. "How long have you been here?" she asked.

"About a week," I said.

"Only a week, and already you can take care of patients?"

"Yes, well, I also had some training at Stanford University Hospital before I came here," I said as I exaggerated my level of expertise.

"Are you in medical school?" she asked.

"I'm starting in the fall." Again, I found myself twisting the answer to my advantage.

She blushed and stammered as she spoke. "I want to go to medical school. But it's really hard to get in." Perhaps I could have encouraged her, but I stood by silently as if to add an exclamation to her statement. I was enjoying the distinctions between us that she was defining, feeling as if my week at the clinic entitled me to it.

We continued sorting medicines as Carl packed a mule and trotted off to a village several hours away to visit a family with a sick child. At least that is what he said, though I suspected he had created an excuse to leave, because he seemed so flustered when the girls had arrived. I was happy to be in charge, suddenly aware that since Dr. Silva had left to go back to the United States, there was no one else. Being in charge meant I could lead the girls around on a variety of orientation tours.

After we had organized the medicines and as I tried to think of something for us to do, a tall, thin man rushed through the clinic door. He had a dark, angular face with eyes that tilted slightly toward his hooked nose. His forehead dripped sweat as he explained how his wife was trying to deliver their baby and had been pushing and cramping for a day and a night. He was frightened that she might die if we didn't do something soon. My first reaction was to explain that I could not help because I had never even seen a baby delivered and to send for Carl. But when I asked Luis if he could get Carl, he shook his head. "He's too far by now." The girls looked at me attentively, and I remembered Carl's advice about reading the books. I even convinced myself that maybe after one week I could do some good. Why else would Carl leave me in charge?

"*Bueno*," I said as I explained the man's story to Katherine and Linda. "I think there's some equipment under the medicine shelf." I pointed to a basin with forceps. I had no idea how to use them. I opened a book about obstetrics and read about prolonged labor. The book said that sometimes a cesarean section might be needed to save mother and child. I began to call for scalpel, retractors, and suturing material, everything I might need. I doubt that I would have actually attempted a cesarean section, but I was doing what Carl had recommended—reading the books. And I wanted to be prepared. Perhaps I imagined an obstetrician might appear suddenly, or Carl might arrive and need the equipment. My mind began to race.

"Luis!" I shouted. He was outside talking with friends, and I waited for him to walk in. "This man's wife is having trouble with her pregnancy. Can you drive me to her?" I thought that maybe with the Jeep we could at least transport the woman to a hospital or back to the clinic.

Luis conversed with the man for a few minutes before answering me. "He lives in Carisol. The Jeep cannot pass there. You need a horse. This man can take you there."

"Where can I get a horse?" I asked.

"Maybe Ricardo will lend us one," he said.

"And see if you can get one for . . ." And I hesitated, looking at Katherine and Linda. I wanted company and thought that having a woman along might be helpful because I had never performed a pelvic exam.

They looked at each other, and Katherine nodded. "OK, I'll go."

"See if you can get one for Katherine," I said.

Luis winked at me and ran off to find horses. The man with the pregnant wife accompanied him, leaving me alone with Katherine in the clinic.

"Have you ever delivered a baby?" Katherine said. For a moment the enormity of what she was asking paralyzed me, and I hesitated. But then, as I felt the admiration and confidence in her eyes, I became unfrozen.

"No," I said, "but Carl has gone over it with me."

We continued to collect equipment and stuffed it into plastic bags. I was both excited and terrified at the prospect of delivering a baby. I tried to concentrate on the mechanics of childbirth and what I might have to do. If the head was stuck, perhaps I could cut an episiotomy or apply forceps. If labor was too weak, I could give a medicine. If the mother was dying . . . The possibilities were dramatic, but I hoped it would all become clear when I arrived and could examine the woman. What other choice did I have? In my mind, I found myself building a bridge of conditionals: if I could suture a wound, then I could suture an episiotomy; if Carl could deliver a baby and thought I could, then maybe . . . if there was no other choice, then . . . And as I built this tenuous bridge, I ignored the reality that I was so far out from my foundation of knowledge that I stood on the edge of a precipice with the consequences of my actions a swirling torrent of disaster below me.

Luis returned with two horses—actually a horse and a mule. The horse had a gray coat, long gray mane, and muscular shoulders that tensed as I touched them. The mule had a chocolate brown coat with a triangle of white on her forehead. The horse belonged to Ricardo's brother Victor and was reputed to be the fastest horse in the village. The mule belonged to Ricardo and was a calm, easy, safe animal. I mounted the horse, holding the reins tightly in my clenched hands, and watched nervously as the man who had come to request our help hurried off down the road on his mule. Katherine was swinging her leg over the saddle of her mule as I gently squeezed my heels into my horse's flanks to indicate that I was ready to move forward.

The horse moved into a bouncing trot and then a slow gallop as it hurried forward to catch the mule ahead of us. I clutched at the saddle horn as we bounded forward, concentrating on keeping my feet in the stirrups. Children playing by the side of the road grinned and pointed at me as I rode by, and I tried to wave nonchalantly back at them, but my horse was accelerating as it neared the mule, following some kind of competitive urge independent of anything I could do. We rushed past the man and his mule on the road out of town, and I heard the man yell at me but could not understand him. Now the horse accelerated into overdrive, and his ears bent back as he sped along the roadway. As the air rushed past me, I could hear the steady grunts of his breathing. On and on we went as I sat frozen, afraid to move, afraid to fall, mesmerized by the power of the horse at a full-out run. Finally, I pulled back on the reins, hoping to slow him before we passed the turnoff to Carisol, where the pregnant woman lived. The horse resisted and swerved as it tried to guess at my request. Was I trying to turn or slow down? We finally slowed to a trot, then a walk. Katherine and the man galloped up to me and stopped. The mules' hooves kicked up dust from the road into my face, and I sneezed as they came alongside.

"*Salud*," said the man.

"Bless you," said Katherine. "What were you doing? Running the Kentucky Derby?"

Before I could explain, the man behind us pointed to a sandy wash with large trees. We had ridden past it and had to turn around to get back on the correct trail. Having demonstrated his superior speed, my horse was now content to walk behind the man's mule as we stepped over rocks and boulders in the twenty-foot-wide wash. A canopy of trees with broad trunks provided shade from the sun, but there was no water, though I imagined there must be some near the surface to support the trees and dense underbrush. Flies and beetles buzzed around us, landing on the animals we rode. My horse twitched his muscles and switched his tail to chase away the flies.

We reached Carisol after about a half hour. A cluster of three houses made up the central settlement, and a few other houses extended out along the trail. We dismounted and removed the saddlebags containing the medical equipment and an obstetrics book I had packed. A rusted Coke sign marked the house, and as I entered I realized that it also served as a small market; there were cases of soda and canned goods piled in a corner. My feet moved tentatively as I walked, my muscles slowly readjusting from riding. When I first entered the dark bedroom, I could not see anything. I heard panting and moaning and a woman's voice calmly urging and instructing. Gradually, their forms came into focus: a woman on the bed holding her own ankles as she thrust her pelvis forward, sweat bathing her forehead; and another woman, gray hair pulled back into a tight braid, kneeling on the floor. I heard the older woman yelling, "Push, push!" as she encouraged the pregnant woman, who pursed her lips, grimaced, and strained to push. A yellow fluid dripped from the pregnant woman's vagina as the top of the baby's head bulged out.

I stood frozen. I had never seen a naked pregnant woman. Katherine came up to me. "What would you like me to do?" she asked.

"Well, I guess we should unpack our equipment," I said.

She nodded. "OK. I'll take the bags into the other room."

The house had two rooms: a kitchen, which also served as the store; and this bedroom with a large wood-frame bed and a rattan chair. The floor was dirt, and wooden shutters, now closed, marked the openings of two small windows. Gradually I noticed other forms: crouching in the corners of the room were two small children and a heavyset woman in a long dress. They sat silently, like pictures on the wall.

Katherine returned with the forceps, which were two huge metal spoons that could be applied to the baby's head in order to pull it out. That seemed like a good idea if the head was stuck on something. I scanned through the book attempting to figure out what I might be able to do. But all of the diagrams of how to extract a baby were too complicated for me to understand. I returned to the bedroom. I watched the older woman massaging the pregnant woman's belly as she waited for a new contraction. She introduced herself to me with a firm handshake, and I noticed she wore no gloves. "Doña Victoria," she said briefly before she returned to her patient.

The fringe of hair bulging in the woman's vagina began to grow until it was about the size of a grapefruit, and suddenly it popped forward as the woman screamed, and the baby's face appeared. It was a Buddha face—round, serene, otherworldly, and frozen in time and space.

"Push, push!" yelled doña Victoria, and I watched as the body emerged covered with yellow and white slime and blood. More blood followed, but we hardly noticed, as doña Victoria slapped the baby's back until it cried weakly and began to breathe. She cleaned off the slime as she slapped it again, and the cry became louder. The umbilical cord pulsed as blood continued to flow through it. "We have to tie the umbilical cord and cut it," I told Katherine. We found sterile nylon suturing material and tied it around the cord in two places. Then I used the scalpel to cut the umbilical cord. It felt like a thick, overcooked noodle springing from my sharp blade; drops of blood appeared at the cut ends. With the umbilical cord cut, we could examine the baby. Doña Victoria washed and cleaned the yellow slime off the baby and wrapped her in a blanket. "It's a girl," I said to Katherine. "I think." The genital area seemed so swollen I couldn't be sure. Katherine handed me a stethoscope, and I listened to the baby's heartbeat. "It's strong," I said. "I can barely count it. About 140." My stethoscope bell almost covered the baby's entire chest. I picked her up and handed her to the mother, who was now smiling proudly. Doña Victoria tugged on the end of the umbilical cord still protruding from the vagina, and a red, pancake-shaped object appeared at the vaginal opening and then dropped onto the ground with a spurt of blood.

"Is that the placenta?" Katherine asked.

"I guess so," I said. I had never seen a placenta before.

The baby quietly sucked at the woman's nipple while the husband and the others in the room now gathered around the baby to admire her.

I felt relieved that we had been spared the difficult decisions about dangerous procedures that I had never seen. My inexperience might have caused me to do real harm. I also realized how naïve I had been to imagine I could arrive with my bags of equipment and do anything useful. But the family seemed to think that our arrival had somehow hastened the birth. The husband thanked me and wanted to give me money, but I told him the services were free.

"You will be paid in heaven," he said.

As we left the house, doña Victoria was performing some kind of ceremony to protect the baby. It seemed like a baptism as she shook droplets of water onto the baby's head. The other woman, who had been sitting on the floor in the corner, chanted softly and sprinkled more water.

"Wow, that was amazing!" said Katherine as we emerged into the sunlight. Her eyes vibrated with excitement that she could barely contain, and she hugged me as she tried to share the feeling. I reciprocated, and we stood outside the little house, embracing. We were both hot and sweaty, and our bodies smelled. I felt her arms loosen, and she patted my back—a signal that the hug was over—and I released her. I was glad to have her company, to share the experience and the ride home. And I wasn't sure anyone would believe my story without a witness, nor would I trust my own memory. It was all too strange, too dangerous, and too risky.

We remounted our animals and rode back down the wash. Several hawks soared overhead, and I thought about the Cokes back at the house and how I wished I'd asked for one before we left.

"I'm thirsty," I said.

"I am too," she said. "I brought water in my canteen."

"You did?"

"Yeah, my dad made me take the canteen full of clean water for the ride down, and I put it on the mule."

"Well, great. Let's take a drink under that tree," I said, pointing to a tree with a trunk at least twenty feet around.

We shared the canteen, and though the water was warm, it tasted delicious and quenched my intense thirst. The horse and mule stood patiently in the shade, chasing away insects with their tails and munching on the leaves of low-hanging branches. I remember thinking that the place was perfect. I moved toward Katherine, and she smiled. She bent toward me and our lips met, still wet from the water. It happened suddenly, without thought, and I began to regret it immediately. Then the animals began to wander off.

"The horses!" I shouted, pulling away from Katherine. As I ran to grab the saddle of the mule, they bounded farther away, down the wash. We chased them, stumbling over the rocks until they were out of sight.

"We lost them," I said.

Katherine shrugged. "I guess we can walk back."

We struggled over the sand and rocks of the wash for almost an hour. My thoughts alternated between Katherine and how we could get back the animals and all our medical equipment that was attached to the saddle. I felt that I should say something, but my thoughts were jumbled, so I just walked.

As we made slow progress, the trees and rocks all began to resemble each other. None of the countryside looked familiar. Slowly a feeling of uncertainty and fear began to build inside my stomach.

Then Katherine stumbled on a root and plunged forward onto the sand. As I helped her up, she favored her right ankle. "I think I twisted it," she said.

"Do you want to rest?" I asked.

She nodded. "I'm really sorry about this."

I looked at her ankle. On the outside near the bone, it was beginning to swell. I pressed on it gently.

"Ouch," she said.

"Sorry," I said. "It's kind of swollen." I looked at her long legs stretched out in front of me, smooth and tapered like a model's.

"I'm too tall," she said.

"Why do you say that?"

"Well, boys are afraid of me. That was my first real kiss."

"Really?"

"Except for those little ones on the cheek. But that was my first time on the lips. My parents are Mormon. But anyway, since it was my first kiss, and then we had to run off after the animals, I wasn't sure if it was officially over, or if there was more to it."

"That was about it," I said.

"Oh," she said. We were roasting in the sun and were almost out of water. I could tell she was disappointed, that she had wanted this to be special, like a birthday.

But I felt embarrassed, and the kiss was only a part of it. Everything about the trip to Carisol felt fraudulent, and now we sat lost among the snakes and scorpions. I felt myself spiraling downward into guilt and despair as I imagined this, my punishment, and realized that it was her first kiss—and not a very good one.

Then I heard animals trotting up to us and saw them kicking sand and pebbles into the air. Ricardo and Tony were looking down from our lost animals.

"When the horse and mule returned without you, we got worried," said Tony. "Ricardo was afraid you or the gringita might have fallen off."

"No, we lost them when we were taking a drink," I said. "And Katherine sprained her ankle when we were walking back. It's swollen. I don't think she can walk on it."

They dismounted to more closely examine the ankle.

"Very well," said Ricardo. "You and the gringita mount the mule, and Tony and I will ride together on the horse." He hoisted Katherine onto the saddle. I jumped on behind her.

When we arrived back at the village, I found crutches for Katherine, and she started to hobble around on the road in front of the clinic. But the crutches were too small, and she stumbled. Linda decided they should begin driving back to the United States to see a doctor.

"You should wait till the morning," I said.

"No," Linda said, "my dad's a doctor, and I know this is broken."

I waved to them as the van departed in a cloud of dust. The suddenness of their arrival and departure had the feel of a dream.

"They're angels," said Loli as he stood with Ricardo and a crowd of other men watching the gringitas disappear down the road. "Angels from God."

"Yes," said Ricardo. "That's why they cannot stay here."

Carl returned the next day. He seemed relieved that the girls had already gone. When I told him about the birth, he did not get angry, as I had anticipated he would. "Doña Victoria is a good midwife. She's delivered half the babies in the village," he said. "Now you've seen a delivery, and next time you will know how to do it." He tried to convince me that I had made the right decision to go and that by just being there, I was helping. Except that next time I should also send Luis to get him in case extra help was needed. But no harm had been done. The family was happy, and I had learned something.

Carl could see the doubt in my eyes and the wrinkles on my forehead, and he bent low and whispered something into my ears—words that made no sense.

"Soon you'll be running the clinic," he said and grinned at me through his beard before walking off.

Chapter Six

AS THE DARKNESS ENVELOPED THE HOUSE IN ALBUQUERQUE, I decided to take a walk. The rooms seemed unfamiliar. Shadows and misplaced chairs created an unexpected set of obstacles.

"Shit!" I shouted as I bumped into a stool and knocked it over. I couldn't remember putting it there in the hall, and I wondered if Laura had moved it. I could turn on some lights and make my walk easy, but I enjoyed the challenge and the misery the darkness created, a punishment that I could blame on Laura if I did get hurt.

I kicked a ball that was lying in the living room. It was Ethan's basketball. I wondered why it wasn't in his room. He was at camp, so I couldn't blame him. Maybe Laura had taken it out when she was packing boxes, to bounce it on the brick floor the way Ethan did.

And then I stepped on the dog, curled up and sleeping near the door. "Oh, Chamisa, poor thing," I said as I tried to pet her and reassure her that I intended no harm. I opened the heavy front door and noticed the stars visible through the gaps between the branches of the huge cottonwood tree in the front yard. I doubted that whoever planted it next to the house fifty years ago had realized what a hazard it would become. As the tree grew bigger and bigger, the wind would tear at the large branches, causing them to crash down onto the roof and walls of our home.

I decided to walk down the road and along the irrigation ditch. I wasn't sure where I was going. I needed some air, and the fresh evening breeze felt comforting. I followed the dirt path past neighbors' houses, peering into windows as I passed, wondering who was fighting, who was watching TV, who was making love. What do we know about other people's lives? What happened behind closed doors was a mystery until some event suddenly revealed it all. Like when Laura moved out and packed up the furniture and boxes. Suddenly we were exposed, our marriage available for dissection by anyone who cared to discuss it. But before that, what did anyone know? We seemed like any other couple, with our grocery shopping and soccer games and morning rush for school and work, our dog barking at passing strangers.

I followed a side trail past a different street, and a dog barked behind a wall. I hurried past and now realized where I was headed. I was on the way to Laura's apartment. It was close enough that the kids would be able to walk between the two homes. I should have called her to let her know, but now it was too late. And anyway, I sort of wanted to look things over first from a distance before I went in. I wanted to see what it looked like and if she had any visitors.

I entered the apartment complex of small separate houses or duplexes. One or two bedrooms. Hers was number 123. Easy to remember. My legs began to shake as I got close. What if someone was there? A man perhaps.

I found 101. Then 115, then 123. The lights were on, and the curtains closed. I heard music coming from the stereo.

She was playing Brian Eno, one of those weird instrumentals that was meant to suggest an environment like a desert or another planet. I remembered she would put it on sometimes in our bedroom after we made love, to help her drift off to sleep. It had that peaceful kind of feel.

I walked up to the door and knocked. She opened it.

"Oh, hi," she said. I noticed she was alone.

"Hi," I said. "I wanted to see your place."

"Oh, fine. Come in."

I looked around. She had already unpacked the boxes and hung pictures. It looked well put together, unlike my house. The lamps were plugged in and shining light in the right places. The stereo worked. The kitchen was clean, and there were no dishes in the sink. I noticed the paintings on the walls, the same ones that had been hanging on our walls a few days before. And the chair with the reading lamp seemed quite comfortable in its new location. Even the books were already in bookcases, organized by topic. There was a travel section, an art section, and a fiction section.

"Looks nice," I said.

"Thanks," she said. "Would you like some tea?"

As she brewed the tea, I watched her. She moved with the same awkward grace I remembered, but now I noticed it more. Her light brown hair was cut short and was combed up away from her forehead.

"How are you doing?" she asked.

"OK."

"You sure looked tired this morning."

"Yeah, I was wiped. But I'm better now. I was looking through the photo album. Some of my Mexico pictures. Some photos of the kids."

"Aren't they cute?"

"Yes. I wonder how they're doing at camp," I said.

"Oh, I'm sure they're fine."

We looked at each other silently for a while, until the kettle whistled.

"What would you like?" she said

"I don't know. Maybe some Good Earth herbal tea."

"OK," she said.

We took our tea and sat down in the two chairs. She had been reading, and I noticed the book was a novel with a tree and a woman on the cover.

"So," I said, "I guess this is it."

"Yes," she said.

"I never thought we'd end up this way," I said.

"Well, nothing is decided. This is just what I need now."

"But why? Why do you need this? We have our house. This will be so hard. And once we start down this road, who knows where it will take us. We can't afford two houses."

"Well, I've been thinking about this for a long time. Years."

"Years?"

"Yes. I didn't tell you, but it's been years."

"Why? What did I do?"

"No, it wasn't you. Not really. I think I'm just not meant for marriage. For living with someone. It's so suffocating. I can't take it anymore. And it's not fair to you. You talk about traveling, about Mexico, about adventure, but deep down, you want a stable routine that repeats itself day after day, with the same work, the same shopping, the same exercise. I can't do that anymore."

"Why not? That's how we live. That's what pays the bills and the kids' school. I do it because I have to for you and them. Sure, I'd like to travel, or go back to the clinic or some other clinic and volunteer and really make a difference for people, but we have this life here that we can't abandon," I said. "And when we have to support two houses, we'll have even less time to do anything else."

"We'll find a way," she said.

"I . . . I don't know," I said.

We sipped our tea and pondered for a while.

"So, if you were feeling this way for years, how could you tell me you loved me?"

"I did."

"And now?"

"I don't know. Maybe I fell out of love. All I know is that I need to be on my own. Make my own way. I need to prove to myself I can do it. When we met, I was only twenty-two. You were older. You had already lived on your own. I hadn't."

"Hell, in Mexico, they get married at fifteen."

"Yes, and in Mexico, women die in childbirth and college students practice medicine."

"It was better than nothing," I said.

"There you go again. I'm sure you did a fine job. But that was Mexico. And that was twenty years ago. I'll bet it's all changed."

"Well, I'm going back there and I'll see. I'm so tired. These night shifts wear me out. And the ER is getting more and more difficult. Every problem that can't be solved ends up there: the lady whose wheelchair breaks, the man whose oxygen tank runs out of oxygen, the drunk who falls asleep in the park, and the baby whose mother is a heroin addict. I can't solve their problems. And then we get the real emergencies: the heart attacks, stabbings, and car crashes. I can't solve them either. I don't think I have it in me anymore. I don't think I can do it all without you. It's too much."

"Oh, you can. You still enjoy it. I can tell by your stories and the excitement before a shift."

"It's not excitement. It's terror."

We finished our tea. I put the cup in the sink. She walked me to the door, and there was that awkward moment when I wasn't sure whether to kiss her or what. She gave me a hug, and I said, "Bye."

I walked back along the ditch and heard the barking dog again. I wondered how I got to this place and imagined rolling back time and changing something. But then I would have to go back years. I wondered when she began to feel this way. And I wondered what I could have done. Perhaps the marriage was meant to come out this way. Perhaps we were never meant to marry or have kids, and we changed our fate through determination and willpower but couldn't sustain it. I wondered if I had really peered inside myself the way she was doing, and if I understood my nature. Or had I just been too busy following a path that was in front of me?

When I got home, I turned on the lights. The furniture was all over the place in odd spots, and books were in piles on the floor. If our houses reflected our inner states, it was clear who was more put together.

I went to the refrigerator for a beer. Even though I had just woken up and eaten breakfast, my body wanted to return to bed, and the beer would ease me in that direction. I enjoyed the rich, almost sweet taste of it over my tongue and down into my throat. I might even have another and put on some music—something mellow, maybe Keith Jarrett, or maybe Dylan. I started humming the tune from a Dylan song: "She makes love just like a woman . . . but she breaks just like a little girl."

The photo album lay out on the table, and I was drawn to pictures from my time in Mexico. There was one picture of a young girl on her mother's lap, her eyes bloodshot and swollen, her mouth half open, caught in the midst of a cough. She was one of our patients from the whooping cough epidemic. We had saved her and perhaps changed her destiny. Who could say what is supposed to be, and memory can play tricks, connecting or disconnecting events. But I felt sure that this little girl was alive with her own children because of what we did during the epidemic.

The epidemic began like a gathering snowstorm. I'd been in the village a few weeks. Cough, cough, cough, cough, cough, cough and a whoop as air refilled the empty, hungry lungs, like the swirl of wind from gray billowing clouds. Cough, cough, cough, cough, cough— whoop—cough, cough, cough, cough, cough—whoop—and then vomit spilled out with the terrible force of spasms of the stomach and chest muscles.

When the patients first arrived, Carl handed out red cough syrup. I heard the coughing spasms as they sat in the waiting room and noticed that the waiting room was full of mothers holding babies and toddlers. Then the people in the waiting room overflowed out into the street. Tony drove to the city to buy more cough medicine and vaccine, and Carl showed me a chapter in a book about whooping cough. He pointed to the symptoms: "spasms of cough," "character-istic whoop at the end of the spasm," and "the mortality rate may be 10–20 percent."

"This is very serious," he said. "We could lose twenty or thirty children."

"Can't we vaccinate them?" I asked, realizing that he and I were protected by our childhood vaccinations. It was a disease we rarely encountered in the United States because vaccination had mostly eliminated it. But here in rural Mexico, vaccination campaigns had not yet arrived and only the fortunate families that had sought out the vaccine from private clinics in the city were protected.

"It's probably too late. The epidemic is here already. I've sent Tony to Mexico City, but he won't be back for a week, and it will probably be too late by then. I wanted to do that last year, but we couldn't get the vaccine. We could have prevented this. But now we have to go house to house and check every child. The book says antibiotics can help if given early." His eyes glowed with excitement as he spoke.

"OK," I said.

"What?" he said, distracted from deeper thoughts.

"OK." I repeated my response.

"Yes. Good. We'll need everyone working together. No time for sleep or food. If you need sleep, you better get it now."

"Now?" I asked, because it was the middle of the day.

He was looking out toward the mountains and did not answer. Then he began writing furiously on a paper: columns, squares, lines, and crosses. Finally he stopped and smiled. "Send them all home," he said. "They're just infecting each other here in the waiting room. Send them home, and tell them I'll see them in their houses. Tell them not to worry." And he showed me his plan. But before I could ask him what it meant, he made new slashes and dashes, added circles, made new arrows, and then folded the paper and slipped it into his jeans pocket. His fingers trembled as he folded the paper, and his lips grimaced, revealing crooked yellow teeth. Droplets of sweat formed at his scalp line, but he had no time for them, and he stood up on his toes as he raced from medicine shelf to medicine shelf counting out doses of antibiotics.

I walked into the waiting room and made the announcement. I explained about the danger of staying in the clinic, assuring them that don Carlos would visit them in their homes. But no one moved. I wondered if it was my Spanish. I tried again, spoke slower and louder, and used different words. A baby had a coughing spasm and a whoop. I pointed to the baby as an example, and the mother plunged the child's head under her dress against her breast. But no one moved. I returned to Carl and explained the situation. He sighed and barely looked at me as he hurried into the waiting room. As he spoke, two children coughed and whooped. He explained his concern again and promised visits, but in the end they all paraded through to have him touch them with his stethoscope and to receive a bottle of medicine.

"They've traveled eight hours on muleback," he'd say as he handed out the antibiotics.

"They took a bus for four and a half hours," he'd say as he handed out another bag of medicine.

And on and on, until we had examined all of them.

"This is what it's all about," he said.

"But what about your plan?" I asked.

"You don't need a plan when you're drowning. You just keep moving your arms and legs until you either make it to land or you die."

My job was to gather up the medicines and write it all down—where the people came from, how many children, what ages. Luis helped by explaining the treatments, answering questions, and ushering the families out as Carl hurried from patient to patient.

At night, the whoops and answering whoops reminded me of an eerie birdsong. I stumbled over the cobbled road with my flashlight and bag of medicines as Carl directed me to the new, untreated cases. Inside a house, the strong smell of herbs and medicinal tea would lead me to the tiny patient lying in the arms of an anxious parent. I'd have to step over relatives lying on the floor who barely budged, and I'd smell the sweat and urine embedded in the canvas cots. Carl spoke to me with animated, wild exhortations to keep going. He asked my opinion and complimented me on my efforts. "We're winning this battle," he'd say and grin at me. "Still no deaths. Just keep it up a few more nights, and we'll be through the worst of it." He took pictures and drew in a notebook so that he could include this in his next fund-raising speech in the United States. I began to understand why the clinic existed, why people donated money and volunteered. He burned with a purpose consuming everything around him, unstoppable, awesome. It was why I had been drawn to that village, to him.

"Too bad Tony's gone," I said. "This could have been part of his movie."

"Yes," he said dreamily.

Several nights later Carl, Luis, and I sat together in the clinic staring at the lists of children we had treated. We were exhausted from the nights of emergency visits and knocks on our door. Carl made jokes and tried to make us laugh.

"*Nalgón.*"

"*Huevón.*"

They cast insults like two adolescents joking and competing, with a familiarity that surprised me. But I was an observer and not a participant as the verbal jousting continued.

"*Préstame.*"

"*Sus nalgas.*"

And they laughed. And I laughed too, because we were a team and needed to laugh together. But I knew I was missing something in the interchange, something that had nothing to do with me. It was strange to watch him with Luis as they tickled and poked each other. A tickle on the stomach and the cheek. I felt awkward about their closeness and playfulness and tried to laugh. But as my eyes met Carl's, I could tell he was probing for my real reaction. And I tried to hold his gaze, match his smile, share, but the intensity in his look made me shudder, and the corner of my cheek twitched as I looked down at the table and the list. His was the look of a poker player, and he knew I was bluffing at his game.

The next day the epidemic was gone. There were no whoops, no new cases. Carl retreated into his books, away from the other patients who visited the clinic, and stared off at distant mountains. I wanted to celebrate, to sing, to yell at the top of my lungs a victory cry, but

Carl would have none of it. I had witnessed his heroism, the reason he was worshipped and trusted by everyone in the village, but he seemed to take no joy in it. The life-and-death struggle and the daily adversity had energized him. Success bored and embarrassed him. He was already off on his next project, a book for medical assistants. Grateful families brought eggs, chickens, and goats, yet he retreated into his loft, leaving me to accept their thanks.

When the gifts stopped coming, he returned to the consultation room and began treating patients again. But he was different—moody, morose, and distant. A crystalline frost seemed to cover him, and the connection between us became weak and tentative.

"Is there something . . . did I do something wrong?" I said finally, because it was so different.

"What? Why, no. You were quite helpful, but now we must return to our regular schedule. There is so much we need to do. So much that I must do."

I had felt a camaraderie and closeness developing as we worked together. But now it was over. He was absorbed in other thoughts, other projects, and I was not a part of them.

Something between us had blown away in the swirling storm of the whooping cough epidemic. I felt a mixture of regret and relief as Carl retreated into the shadows.

Chapter Seven

I FELT A DULL NUMBNESS IN MY HEAD AS I SAT IN MY DIM house in Albuquerque drinking beer after beer. But all the sweetness was gone from the beer. The last sip tasted stale and metallic, and my head felt numb with the first sensation of drunkenness. I replayed my conversation with Laura. All those years she had been struggling and hiding it from me. It was too painful. I drifted back to Mexico, and let myself continue along the trail of reconstructed memories, filling in details as I closed my eyes and rubbed them with my fingers.

I thought back to the whooping cough epidemic and our heroic actions. We had saved children who would surely have died. But after that, everything seemed to get more complicated. I thought back to those days after the epidemic, and what had happened still made me shake my head in amazement.

After the whooping cough epidemic, I began to see my own patients, asking for help with Spanish or medicine as I needed it. Carl encouraged it. "That's how you learn," he said. We reviewed the library of donated books. "You can start with *Differential Diagnosis*. It tells you what diseases cause what signs or symptoms. Then you move on to *Current Therapeutics* and find what medicine you give for the most likely diagnosis. It's really quite simple."

"What if you're not sure, even after reading the books?" I asked. "I mean, for headache the book talks about brain tumors and meningitis and also migraines. One problem might kill the patient and for the other, you can give aspirin. How do you know which it is?"

"You can never be sure," he said. "So you try something, and if it doesn't work, you try something else. We have a whole roomful of medicines."

And then something occurred to me that I had neglected to ask when I had considered it previously.

"Well, don't people here in Mexico have to go to medical school and take tests to do what we're doing? I mean, can anyone just go out and be a doctor? Wouldn't that be dangerous? I mean, couldn't I get into trouble?"

"Oh, the government knows what we're doing here. I have a letter of commendation from the president of Mexico. They can't get a doctor to practice here, and even the program for mandatory rural medical service hasn't been able to send anyone here. No, we are all they have. Maybe someday one of our boys from the village will go to medical school and come back here. I keep hoping that by setting an example, we will inspire someone to do it. We'll even help pay for it. But for now, you and I are their best choice and their only choice."

I nodded, and he smiled at me—a strange smile, as if he had now shared an important secret for which I should be grateful. And there was not a trace of concern for a mistaken diagnosis or wrong treatment.

I followed his procedures. My patients didn't seem to mind that I read books as I treated them. Everyone left with a small bottle of medicine because I always had some diagnosis, and each diagnosis had a suggested therapy in the book. And no one seemed to complain or suffer from a wrong treatment. A week later, when Carl told me he had to leave for a few weeks, I felt confident that I had a good system that worked. "I have to give a speech for the foundation's fund-raiser, and then we have a meeting of the foundation's board of directors," he said.

"What's the foundation?" I asked.

"It's the way the clinic gets money, tax deductible. If you give enough money, you get on the board."

"Oh, I wondered how we could give out medicine without anyone paying."

"Well, that's only a small part. There's the building and the Jeep and gas for the generator and trips like this one. We are very frugal here because every penny is precious."

"Oh," I said. "Well, I'll try not to waste anything or let anyone die."

"Don't worry. You'll do fine." He patted my shoulder and smiled. "I go back and forth to the United States three or four times a year to bring down donated medicine, and I leave the clinic empty. You'll be much better than an empty clinic."

Later that day, I watched him drive away with a sense of excitement and dread. That night, I tossed and turned, worrying about my sudden elevation to doctor of the village. I wondered if the foundation's board would have approved. Carl seemed to mistake my eagerness to learn for competence. I never let on how frightened I was or how I worried about making the right diagnoses. Perhaps he saw in me a validation of his theory that anyone could cure illness with a few books and some shelves of medicines. And I believed him. I wanted him to believe in me. I realize now that I was fortunate that the villagers believed in the will of God and the relative powerlessness of medicine to change it.

I was asleep when a man came for me. "Oiga, oiga, oiga, David! It's my son. He is very sick."

"OK, let me get dressed." As I got out of bed, Rosa appeared with a flashlight for me, shaking her head. I put on my clothes and met the man, don Felipe, at the clinic. His son was breathing rapidly. He was Gerónimo, the músico who had played at the latrine-building project and at the dance. I remembered him and something about his diabetes.

"Diabetes?" I asked them.

"Yes," said don Felipe.

"Has he been taking his insulin?"

"Yes." They looked at each other and nodded.

I looked in my books and read about diabetes. As long as he was taking his insulin, I didn't have to worry about the most feared complication, ketoacidosis. But diabetes could also lead to infections like pneumonia. That must be it. I listened to the lungs, and they seemed congested.

"Pneumonia," I announced triumphantly. "Here, take these antibiotics and you should be better in a few days."

"Doctor, could he have an injection?"

"Sure," I said. "I will give him an injection, and he can sleep in the clinic tonight. Then I'll give him another tomorrow."

"Thank you, Doctor," said don Felipe, his small moustache

twitching. "My son is not very smart. But he loves his music. He is very special to us."

"Don't worry; he'll be fine," I answered.

As I prepared the injection of penicillin, the músico began to sing a beautiful mournful tune: "*Voy a cantar un corrido d'un amigo de mi tierra, llamado se Valentín que fue fusilado y colgado en la sierra.*"

"Tell him to save his breath," I said.

"He sings when he is frightened."

I gave the injection and left to the sound of more singing. "*No me quisiera acordar que era una tarde de invierno, cuando por su mala suerte . . .*"

A few hours later, while it was still dark, I decided to check on him. Perhaps it was the quiet that bothered me. With my flashlight, I made my way to his cot. The light bounced off his eyes, and I knew. They stared straight up, motionless, up to the stars. White vomit covered his mouth. I cried out. Don Felipe, who had been sleeping next to him, jumped up and began wailing and moaning. Somehow, the village awakened, and people began to appear at the bedside. First, two relatives; then some musician friends. Candles and lanterns appeared.

"I'm sorry," I said.

"Oh, no," said don Felipe. "This was the will of God. I knew he would take my son soon. He needed him to play the music in heaven." And he collapsed, crying, against two musicians who had begun to sing.

They lifted Gerónimo onto a cart, and we walked down the road in a procession as musicians played their instruments and sang, while friends and relatives cried and asked God why.

It was not the peaceful moment of wisdom and contemplation that I had thought it would be, this first death of a patient of mine. Instead, it was a moment of horrific, nightmarish terror. Unexpected, sudden, and terrible. And his expression—the eyes that would not close and the mouth in a frozen gape of unbelief. Nothing in my books had prepared me for it, and I found myself wondering and wondering what I had done.

Tony appeared with his camera. "This is incredible," he said, as he filmed the procession. "This is how I want to die. He was doing what he loved, singing his songs. And now his music is all around him."

I stared at him, speechless, as he pointed his camera from the mourners to the musicians. The voices of musicians fluttered into the air, crying out about lost lovers, and I imagined them fusing with the lonely voice of the músico as he had sung—with arms flailing wildly and eyes turned toward the heavens. Then Tony pointed his camera at me, and I put up my hands.

"This is not a movie," I said, still trying to grapple with the reality of my fallibility. I wondered if I had read more, checked on him sooner, done something differently, it might have changed what happened. There would be no chances to try other medications, and the músico was not an actor pretending to be dead. "It's not a movie," I said again.

Chapter Eight

I DIDN'T WANT TO THINK ABOUT MEXICO ANYMORE. I grabbed the photo album to look at the pictures of my children. They were blowing out candles at their birthday parties, climbing rocks, holding the dog, playing soccer or basketball, or riding a horse. My daughter, who knew exactly how to get what she wanted from me, with her dark brown eyes, chestnut hair, and voice a violin to my ears; and my son, with curly hair and sunshine smile, always asking questions when a decision did not suit him. Fortunately, they were at camp, but they knew what was going on—that Mom wanted her own house, that they would be living in two houses. Tears welled up in my eyes as I thought about them and how all this would change their world forever and how I would have done anything to have avoided it. I paged back to photos of my parents young and in love at their wedding. How had they stayed together all these years? Their friends had all stayed married too, for more than forty-five years, while all of mine were breaking up after ten, twelve, fifteen years. I closed the album and decided to go back to bed to escape the painful thoughts and refresh my tired legs, neck, and back, but it was no use. I couldn't stop thinking about Mexico, that first death, and what I learned after it. How they all looked to me, trusted me. I slept fitfully that night.

As I reviewed the details of the músico's death, I realized that I never should have been in that position. Someone with more experience would have recognized the rapid breath and the smell of ketosis and would have given insulin. Someone with more than two weeks of experience. All the books and effort could not replace the experience of seeing the breathing pattern and dehydration of ketoacidosis. If I had only known then what I know now, the músico would have lived. Now, memories of so many diseases—meningitis, measles, diphtheria—inhabit the recesses of my mind, ready to display themselves when a matching patient appears before me. It happens in an instant of recognition when I walk into a patient's room and notice the lips are not right or maybe the eyes, and without thinking, I know. But back then, I knew nothing. And I did not even realize it.

Carl should have known what could happen. Even though no one blamed me, the memory continued to haunt me for years. And Carl should have protected me or prepared me. I suppose he was busy driving twenty hours nonstop to California and raising money. And the only other American was busy capturing the events on film.

After he had filmed the death procession, Tony turned to me. "Hey, man, I didn't mean to hassle you. I just got excited when the shot came along. In the dark, with the lanterns and torches. It was perfect. You know what I mean?"

"I don't know. I guess so. You know, he was alive a few hours ago, singing, and now . . ."

"Was he the same musician at the clinic that day when I was filming the digging?"

"Yes."

"Great," he said. "I have a whole story on film."

Then he paused for a while and put his arm around me. "Hey, sorry, man. You did your best."

"I don't know. Maybe a real doctor would have figured out what to do. If Carl had been here . . ." We lapsed into silence for a minute. I realized that we all used Carl Wilson's first name when we talked about him, except villagers, who called him don Carlos or Doctor. He preferred Carl, but I still felt awkward when I said it.

"Carl's not so perfect either. He makes mistakes too."

"What do you mean?" I said.

"Well, I've seen him make mistakes. I mean that the guy makes you feel like he knows everything, but he doesn't. I first met him when I was thirteen. I told you he was like a big brother. Actually, he was my teacher. My favorite teacher. He was like another kid, but better. He taught me about cameras at camp. He would joke with me, wrestle, and play games. My parents were in the middle of splitting up. He was the first adult who seemed to care about me. We went into the darkroom to develop our pictures. It was so dark in there. Darker than tonight. At first I thought it was sort of like when you bump into someone in the dark. Some kind of game. You just put out your hands and feel your way around, and you never know for sure what you're touching and who's touching you. That's the secret of dark places."

"So what happened?" I asked.

"Everything," he said.

"Everything," I said.

I stood there speechless. It must have been ten, fifteen years ago. Tony described it calmly, as if it was nothing serious.

"What did you do?"

"Nothing," he said. "I didn't tell anyone. I mean, what do you say? When you're a kid, what do you do? Who do you tell? Anyway, he said not to tell anyone because they wouldn't understand, and we'd get in trouble."

I thought about it for a minute.

"Do you think Luis . . . ?" I hesitated now that the answer seemed obvious.

He smiled. "What do you think? Even though they keep it pretty quiet, all the signs are there. Maybe I can see them because I've been there. Haven't you ever seen Luis in the morning at the clinic? He sleeps in the loft with Carl."

Now it all made sense to me. That first night when Luis and Carl disappeared to sleep. The strange intimacy between them. I had imagined it was an innocent kind of friendship, even the playful pokes and hugs, even as it made me uncomfortable.

Now I felt stupid and confused. Stupid because I missed this obvious relationship and confused because no one else seemed bothered by it. And I had even been jealous of the relationship and my exclusion from it.

"What about Luis's parents? Do they know?" I said.

"They're probably just happy that he can visit the United States, and they don't have to feed him or pay for his school," he said. "So they ignore it. Like everyone else."

"And you're still friends with Carl?"

"Yeah," he said. "He's been there for me when I needed someone.

He still cares about me, but not that way. It's just his thing, and it's a little weird, but that's what I mean. He ain't perfect either."

I didn't know what to say. Tony seemed so matter-of-fact, without any anger or blame. For a moment I even wondered if it was true, or if he was joking. But I knew it was true. I wondered what to think of Carl. And what about Luis? And were there others? If Tony had told me about this so that I would feel better about my own mistakes, he had failed. I felt worse: abandoned and disillusioned.

I had wanted Carl to stand for something I could strive toward. But now I began to question everything about him. Was his presence in the village to help people or was it to find a safe place to attract boys like Luis? He was devoting his life to this poor village, and he had created something that worked, that saved lives. And he did all this without concern for wealth. He did it alone, without a wife or family. He was like the holy man who had made a vow of poverty and traveled the world doing good deeds for spiritual enlightenment. And I had wanted to follow him. To be like him. I wanted to know that helping others could be enough, that we weren't all out for ourselves, that you didn't have to get rich out of people's suffering.

When I was growing up, I remember my parents pointing in awe at the beautiful homes where doctors lived. But it was awe mixed with anger.

"That's where Dr. Benton lives," they'd say. "Thinks he's better than the rest of us." My dad would tell me the story of the fight he once had with a doctor, over a girl. "I punched him in the nose. Knocked some sense into him. Now he's head of orthopedics at Massachusetts General Hospital."

I wanted to be the kind of doctor who could inspire awe, but also one whom my parents would still love. Carl had seemed like someone who could help me figure out how to do that. If he could not be my role model, who could? Tony's story made me wonder about myself and whether anyone was motivated by a desire to help others, or if there was always a hidden selfish goal. It could be money or a beautiful woman, or young boys. These basic human moral failings must be the natural result of too much money or power or uncontrollable desire.

Tony explained. "He helped me become a filmmaker. Paid for courses. Sent me to film camp. Hey, he was OK."

I sighed. I wanted to tell him I was sorry for what had happened to him, but he didn't seem to want my sympathy. He looked at the frown on my face and continued. "You don't have to worry. He likes 'em younger—eleven, twelve, thirteen, maybe up to eighteen. You're safe." He smiled.

Eleven, twelve, thirteen. How old had Tony been? Thirteen? How many others were there? What did Carl do with them? One moment I wanted to know everything, and the next, I wanted to know nothing, to blot it out and make it disappear. Today, as an emergency physician, my course would be clear: call the police, get help for the children, remove Carl from contact with children. There were pedophile priests, teachers, and doctors, and no amount of power or reputation could stop the police investigation. That's the protocol for child sexual abuse in emergency departments across the country, and there is no room for gray areas, special situations, or explanations. But at that time, we did not acknowledge or even believe sexual abuse existed. And no one seemed to be complaining; no one was upset. Carl was almost a god worshipped by everyone in the village. You don't arrest a god. And anyway, who would I tell in a little Mexican village? I was already drowning, barely able to breathe between crises, uncertain and trapped. This was just more on top of what I already did not know how to handle.

As Tony and I returned to our homes in the dark, I was blind as I felt my way along the houses and streets, tripping on rocks, feeling for Tony's hand. Dogs barked at us, and I felt one brush by. There were stories of rabid dogs wandering the village at night. One bite could be fatal. As Tony and I groped along, I imagined how the eyes of a rabid dog would melt into this darkness. And I remembered Tony's words, "you're safe." But groping along the irregular stones of the road and the wooden doorposts, I didn't feel safe.

I felt as if I had been dropped into a dangerous world without rules, with a new language. And Carl, who was supposed to be my anchor as I explored this world, had been revealed to me as another piece of the shifting landscape. As I tried to understand Carl, I found myself alternately refusing to believe it—creating excuses—and becoming angry.

I wondered what I would do when he returned. I considered leaving, going back home; but just like Tony and Luis, I still felt drawn to Carl and all he was doing, and so I tried to understand and accept him as Tony had. I didn't want to abandon the villagers just as they were beginning to trust me. I was beginning to feel the immense power of their trust even as I realized I didn't deserve it. It was a power to know hidden details, touch forbidden places, and make pronouncements. It was an intoxicating, dangerous power, and it was part of Carl's world.

Chapter Nine

CARL'S WORLD INCLUDED PEOPLE WHO BELIEVED IN powerful spirits that could cause illness or death and in the intervention of other opposing powers to cure illness. The clinic straddled the spirit world, with its witches, spells, and evil eyes, and another world where tiny microorganisms caused illness, and antibiotics could cure them. Carl seemed to live in both worlds, and perhaps his unusual relationships existed in the space between worlds. I remembered how I had initially thought that I lived in only one world, the world of scientific medicine. I would be guided by scientific methods and combat the dangerous folk beliefs. I didn't know that the same patients who came to the clinic and accepted my bottles of medicine would also consult herbalists and witches for potions and spells.

But I had heard that some people thought Carl was a witch who could control thoughts and people. Perhaps they considered all of us at the clinic a different variety of witch with different powers and bottles instead of spells, but witches nonetheless—witches with strange appetites and desires and great powers. And as I lurched from book to book seeking answers for strange symptoms, I became desperate enough to try anything that might work, particularly if the patient encouraged it, like the small woman with wild eyes who first led me down this path. She wore black, like a grieving widow, her dark eyes peering out from a scarf that covered her head. And she arrived at dusk, as my last patient was leaving the clinic.

"Mañana," I told her. "Come back tomorrow."

"Please, Doctor, I must speak with you." She was insistent. The intensity of her eyes frightened me.

"Pásale." I motioned to her to come in.

We sat down in my office, and she began her story softly, as if afraid that someone might overhear it.

"Doctor, I have a . . . a . . . frog in my stomach."

"A frog?"

"Yes, Doctor, a frog."

I looked for a hint of a smile, wondering if someone was trying to play a cruel joke on me. In this little village, people were always joking and making fun of my Spanish pronunciation. But the woman showed no trace of a smile.

"How do you know it's a frog?" I asked.

"I can feel it."

"Well, but it could be gas in your stomach or maybe a parasite?"

"No, it's a frog. I can feel it jumping. Here, feel it," she said, and she put my hand on her stomach. I searched for a lump or a pulsation or perhaps the movement of gas.

I didn't feel anything. "Well, how did it get there?" I asked.

She stared at me hesitantly, carefully measuring the next sentence. "A witch put it there," she said.

"A witch?"

"Yes, he's my neighbor. He wants my cornfield, but I don't want to sell it to him, so he did this to me."

"Well, I wish I could help you, but we just give out medicines here. And we don't have any pills for your problem," I said.

She looked at me skeptically and began to move away toward the door. Her face remained determined.

"Wait a moment, Señora. I have a question," I said. She turned. "What if you can't get rid of the frog? What will you do?"

"We have to kill the witch. It's the only way, unless I can find some-one with stronger power to take out the frog."

"Um . . . ," I muttered. "So you want me to unbewitch you, to get the frog out?" I asked.

"Yes, Doctor, please. I can't sleep the entire night."

I contemplated the ceremony I might concoct, with chanting and odiferous potions and bits of hair and blood and articles of clothing and smoke and drums. It seemed crazy. I had come to this clinic as a volunteer, to use modern medical techniques to combat superstitions such as this. Yet the possibility intrigued me, and it might save a life.

I looked around the clinic. An empty medicine tin could provide noise. Liniment could provide odor and texture. A dental cotton ball could provide the shape and form to hold or wear. I gathered more equipment—adhesive tape, antibiotic ointment, isopropyl alcohol, and baby powder. All could be useful in my ceremony.

I gathered Deanna and Gabriel as assistants and assigned them tasks—beat the drum, shake the baby powder—while I slathered a wooden tongue blade with liniment and antibiotic ointment. The patient extended her arms to present me with a folded dress that belonged to her, and I carefully applied my smelly ointments to it. Then I walked around her and chanted. "Go away frog," I said while I showered her head and face with baby powder. Round and round I went, like acting in a play, until finally I told her the ceremony was over and that the frog would be gone in the morning. Gabriel helped me clean up and hobbled away on his crutches as if his knee was throbbing.

I slept fitfully that night, dreaming about the frog and then the other witch, but I awakened ready to begin morning hours in the clinic. There would be a line of patients waiting for me. At the front of the line stood the woman. I expected that she would tell me the frog was back, that our treatment had failed, and I had no idea what I would do, because I had already done too much. I asked her how she felt.

"Fine."

"Then why are you here?"

"Well, Doctor, I have a long trip to make, and I am worried the medicine will wear off."

"OK," I said. "It is a very strong medicine, but I will give you something else for the trip."

And I made a small amulet to put around her neck. Inside I enclosed two Valium tablets. "Take this and wear it around your neck. If you feel the frog trying to get back inside you, open the amulet and eat what is inside."

"Thank you, Doctor," she said.

The other patients in line watched her walk away with a tinge of envy in their eyes. It was still early, and she had already been cured.

Chapter Ten

A FEW DAYS AFTER I HAD BROKEN THE WITCH'S SPELL, I HAD my most difficult case. Even today, it would be difficult, if not impossible. The woman in the house had tetanus. The frozen, clenched jaws and the intermittent seizures had pointed me in the right direction, but ultimately it was the Band-Aid attached to the bottom of her foot that had been my clue. "A piece of wood?" her daughter asked. "How could a piece of wood have caused this?"

I tried to explain to the daughter and her husband, who were the woman's only family, how tetanus bacteria entered a wound and produced a poison—a toxin that stiffened muscles in the jaw (lockjaw)—causing the body to convulse and finally raising the body's temperature so high that vital biochemical reactions could not occur and death followed. Treatments were experimental and required intensive care in a hospital. In my broken Spanish, I said, "Hospital. Hospital." They didn't seem to understand. That was when I found Luis and asked him what to do. I told him what I had read in the books and that the woman needed to be in a hospital.

Luis talked to the family, explaining what the books said about tetanus and how the woman would die if she stayed in the village, and that she needed the hospital in Mazatlán with real doctors and intensive care units.

"They told me they want her to stay here," he said. "They trust you. And anyway, they don't have money for the hospital," he said.

"But she'll die here. And anyway, they shouldn't trust me—I'm not a real doctor. I'm just helping Carl."

"Carl is not here," he said.

"So what should we do?" I asked him. I felt strange, posing such a question to Luis, who, at fifteen, was six years younger than I and knew nothing of medical ethics or philosophy. In fact, he could barely communicate without a crude joke or some self-promotion. But he had grown up in the village and had worked with Carl for years.

"Just take care of her. If she dies here, at least the family will be with her, and they won't have to sell their little farm to pay the doctor at the hospital."

"But maybe she wouldn't die if we took her to the hospital."

"Maybe," he said, without any of the weight of the responsibility that the word engendered in me. He smiled as he might have done to cheer up Carl, his eyes bright, his teeth a row of small pale tiles, and for the first time I could understand the attraction between this village boy and the famous philanthropic doctor. His smile expressed acceptance of events beyond our control.

And so we went into the house and set up the intravenous fluids and administered the experimental medicines the way the book recommended. During the next two days, Luis transformed himself before my eyes. I watched as he comforted the family, bathed the woman, told me what I needed to do to prepare everyone for the inevitable death, and walked with me at night through the deserted, unlit streets to make sure I got to bed safely. I would have been lost without him, and it was difficult to admit it—to admit he'd do anything that was not ultimately for himself, that could help me. Ever since learning the nature of his relationship with Carl, I had assumed that was his only dimension.

As we walked home at night, he put a hand on my shoulder. I pulled away.

"What are you doing?" I asked.

"The hole, you were about to step in it."

I looked back at the dark jagged edges of an eroded gully that had carried away a portion of the dirt road. It was not easily visible in the darkness.

"Sorry. I didn't see it."

We walked together in silence for a minute. I did not know what to say, and I felt foolish.

"Thanks for helping me," I said.

"She's a very sick lady. I think she is going to die," he said.

"Yes, but at least we can stop her seizures and let her rest," I said.

"You are starting to be like Carlos," he said. "Sometimes when he would have a patient like this, he would forget to eat or sleep. I would bring him food, so he would eat." And he laughed. "You Americans care for the bodies of others, but forget about your own bodies. Why?" And he smiled. I had no answer.

By the time the woman died, Luis and I had become a team, sharing the hopelessness through a brief glance or a sigh, waiting for the end. Her illness lasted two horrible days, and as we left the family when the final seizure ended, we decided to take a swim in the river to cleanse the sweat, dust, and death from our bodies.

As we walked down to the river, we could finally acknowledge the nightmare of the past two days. *"Muy malo,"* we said as we followed the steep trail down to the swimming and bathing hole.

The men's bathing hole was a deep pool at a bend in the river surrounded by sheer cliff walls that formed a long flat step just before reaching the water. This step created a perfect lounge area for bathers to undress, towel, or just lie in the sun.

When we reached the step, I was surprised we were alone. The heat of the day was unrelenting, and the only escape from it was the river. But most of the men and boys were out tending the cornfields. Luis effortlessly stripped off his clothes and dove quickly into the pool. I was more self-conscious about my nudity, carefully folding my clothes and looking back up the trail.

"Come in!" he yelled at me. And finally I pulled off my underwear and joined him in the pool. It was a sudden, overwhelming feeling to be floating in the cool river water. I became instantly aware of the exhaustion of my muscles and the fatigue of my mind. This death that I had attended had been a continuing torture—no peace, no quiet, no acceptance. But as I floated in the pool, the river water washed it all out of me. Luis frolicked like a ten-year-old, climbing rocks and diving into every spot of the pool. I felt too old for that, but I watched with envy.

Finally I felt cold and climbed back onto the rock step. The sun's warmth felt comforting rather than oppressive as it dried my skin. Luis came over next to me.

"Muy bueno," he said.

"Yes, it's good." I agreed with him.

I looked at his naked body dripping water, and I knew I had to ask him the question that had been bothering me ever since I had learned about his relationship with Carl.

"Luis," I said, "I was wondering about you and Carl." He looked at me, perplexed. "I mean, you sleep with him."

"Well, just sometimes," he said.

"What I mean, I guess, is that I don't understand. I mean, you like girls so . . ."

"Well, Carl wants me to stay with him sometimes. But I think I'm going to stop soon. I'm too old for it."

"But you don't have to do it."

"No, but he pays for my schooling, takes me to California," he said.

"But you shouldn't do it for that."

He paused and looked at me. "Would you help me?"

Attached to his words were the implications of financial support, responsibility, and commitment. His eyes expressed an openness to possibility and challenged me to examine my life and my values. What was I really willing to do? I was completely unprepared. "Sure," I said, but as soon as I said it, I knew I was lying. I wouldn't, couldn't. I knew that Luis and the village would melt away for me when I returned home, to be replaced by medical school, family, a house, and another life. And Luis would have no place in it. I knew that I could offer him nothing. And he knew it too. He looked at me with his accepting smile and forgave me my lie.

Chapter Eleven

AFTER AN UNEASY NIGHT OF DREAMS AND AWAKENINGS, I finally opened my eyes to the bright New Mexico sunlight sneaking through the shades. I had a full day scheduled in the office with meetings and faculty evaluations, and I needed to plan my trip to Mexico if I was really going. The memories of those first weeks in Mexico had suddenly come alive, making me acutely aware of who I had been then—my ideals, my mistakes, and my confusion. And yet, I had pushed forward, certain that the general direction was correct even if the road was twisted. Was I wrong to do that? The clinic was there, and people believed in it. How could you argue with that?

Images of exhausted women breast-feeding crying babies in the waiting room of La Clínica flashed in front of my eyes as I waited for the traffic light to change on my way to work. When horns honked behind me, I realized the light had turned green without my noticing.

When I arrived at my office, my secretary greeted me. "You look tired."

"Yeah, it was a tough night," I said.

"There are travel vouchers to sign and two phone calls to answer, and your first meeting is in ten minutes with residents."

"Residents?" I asked.

"Yes, you are lecturing on medical malpractice."

"Oh," I said. "One of my favorite topics. Fortunately I can wing it because I've done it before."

She smiled. "And Rick said he needs to talk to you."

"Rick? Is it his evaluation?"

"No, he just wanted to discuss something with you. He wouldn't tell me what it was."

"OK," I said. "I've got a little time before the residents, and then it looks like I have a meeting with security." I looked at my appointment card.

"Yes," she said. "I already told him."

I nodded.

Rick came in. His eyes bulged out behind his horn-rimmed glasses, and his beard covered the rest of his face. His brown hair, slicked back over his ears, was more of what I would have expected from a musician than a doctor. He would often surprise people because he looked like a left-wing liberal, but he really was more of an anarchist or a libertarian.

"Are you OK?" he asked.

"Yeah, thanks. And I want to pay you back for those shifts you're doing for my Mexico trip."

Rick smiled, his eyes glowing like a jack-o'-lantern.

"I'll tell you what," he said. "I'm working in the ER tonight, and I just saw Clayton Jones down in our waiting room. What I want you to do if you really want to pay me back is kick him out of the waiting room so I won't have to see him tonight."

"Kick him out? But, Rick, you know we can't do that. He's got sickle-cell anemia. He might be having a sickle crisis."

"Oh, you know Clayton. He sells those Percocets we give him. He got busted a month ago for trying to hire a prostitute by offering her Percocet, and it turned out the prostitute was really a policewoman. He's a drug addict, and we're just feeding his habit."

"But he also has sickle-cell. How can we ever tell whether his pain is real? I mean, would you want sickle-cell? You know he's going to die soon. He's getting up there, for a sickler."

"Yeah, we've been taking care of him for at least fifteen years. When he sees me, he knows I won't give him any morphine or Demerol, so he just sits there and bugs the nurses until they make me give in," said Rick.

"So why don't *you* kick him out?" I asked.

"I don't want to get in trouble with my chairman," he said.

"But I'm your chairman."

"My point exactly," he said and laughed.

"Rick, you know it would be a violation of our policies. It would be illegal, and it would be unethical. I mean, I understand how you feel. I get frustrated when I see Clayton too. But he's almost like family. Most of our patients come once, and we never see them again. But Clayton is a regular. How many times do you think you've seen him?"

"Well, lately it seems like he's coming in more often. I don't know, maybe a hundred."

"That would be six times a year, more or less, for fifteen years."

"Oh, I think it's more than that."

"And figure he tries to avoid you, so you probably see him less than the rest of us," I said.

"Yes, I think he gets our schedule. But you know, we're always trading shifts. I'll bet he comes in when I'm working for you. That's why I want you to kick him out now. Then he won't come in when he sees your name on the schedule even though it'll be me that's working."

"Rick, I think I understand your twisted logic, but I can't do it. Sorry."

"You're such a liberal. Every time I think I've got you coming around to my way of thinking, this sixties liberal shit comes out."

"No, it's just that you are moving so far to the right, that you're coming around to the left. At the extremes, we see the same reality, but you think it's good and I think it's bad. It's those people in the middle who get confused all the time," I said.

"It's just that I believe in survival of the fittest," he said. "We've kept this guy alive all these years, and how many kids does he have? Five, six, and they all carry that sickle gene. And who pays for them all? Who pays for all his visits to the ER and all the times we admit him? He must cost us over a hundred thousand dollars a year. And then we don't have any money to pay for vaccinations for babies from the South Valley because Clayton Jones used it all up and bought prostitutes with his pain pills."

"OK, Rick, you feel better now. I know that deep down you actually like Clayton. I've seen you talking to him. It's just this little game that the two of you play," I said.

Rick grinned. "I guess I've seen Clayton Jones and know him better than most of my friends. I'm gonna miss him, in a way, when he finally dies."

"See, Rick. You really don't want him to suffer or die."

"No, I just don't want you to think I'm an asshole," he said. He laughed and got a smile out of me.

"You know the residents watch how we treat people like Clayton or the chronic alcoholics. So we have to be careful because of the messages we give them too," I said.

"Well, they need to understand the way the world works. If you come in here dressed like a bum and stinking of alcohol and piss, you're going to wait longer than some guy in a tie with a MasterCard in his hand. And if you are a resident, and I ask you to do something, like admit the patient or do a consult, I expect you to do it, no questions asked. If the residents want to fight about it, that's their problem," he said. "But I'm trying to teach them how to survive in the real world. People come to us expecting miracles, and even if we don't have a miracle, we can't be stupid."

"You know, Rick, that in the resident sleep room there is a message board. At the top it says 'Dr. Rick is my daddy,' and they signed it and dated it. There are names going back years."

"Good," said Rick, and he laughed. "I used to think the residents would remember some of the statistics I taught them or the causes of metabolic acidosis. But I'm happy to be their daddy. Remember how no one would respect us when we started? They thought of ER doctors like us as stupid moonlighting interns. The ER was a place no self-respecting specialist would go. And anyone who worked there with the drunks and screaming psychos had to be dumb or desperate. The ER was like a smelly, mosquito-infested swamp. But they didn't realize that it was also the place where all the fish lived, and they would starve without us and our fish."

"Well, it was that, and they'd also look down on us because we could never know as much as they did about their specialties. I mean, how many scleroderma patients do we ever see? Maybe one or two a year. The rheumatologist is bound to know more about what the various anti-DNA tests show. So we seem stupid to them. But they don't realize that we take care of everything that walks in the door or gets brought to us by an ambulance," I said.

"Yeah," he said. "Now that we have our own emergency medicine residents, it's sort of changing. Our residents are our children. Actually, they are better than children because they listen to us. They get to call up the other residents and have those arguments we used to have, and they work out their own rules and punishments for breaking the rules. I can sit back and just be the professor and make stuff up and pimp them with questions that were in the textbooks twenty years ago that they will never be able to answer," Rick said.

"You're plenty smart enough that you don't need to play those pimping power games," I said.

"But it's fun," he said. "It's fun to see their faces turn red when they don't know the answer. Didn't you ever torture grasshoppers when you were a kid? We all did it. They're my little grasshoppers. They're yours too."

"Well, I ask them questions," I said, and I hesitated, considering whether maybe he was right. Maybe I did enjoy asking questions that I had asked many times before and watching the residents and students twist and turn uncomfortably in the silence before I gave the answer. And the smiles and nods of relief afterward. "But not in a cruel, sadistic way."

"Oh, come on," he said. "We all do it. Admit it. And we do it more when there are pretty girls in the audience. I see you looking at them too. We're not as different as you think. Our genes are almost the same as monkeys. We are wired to behave just like them. If we don't, it's because we are fighting our natural feelings. But even with all those years of training and ethics courses and punishments for bad behavior, we still want to be the alpha male with seven or eight wives in our tribe. Luckily, my wife understands. " Rick laughed in another spasm that made his glasses shake on his face and turned to open the door, as if to escape before I could respond.

"Rick, you're a sicko," I said. "You make it sound like we're all on this weird sexual power trip."

"Isn't that why we became doctors?" he said. "For money or sex?"

"No, Rick," I said. But his statement made me pause and think about Mexico and Carl. When people are sick, they don't think about sex, and they'll give whatever money they have in order to get well. Certainly Carl was not interested in money, and he had created a clinic where money barely existed. But sex was a different matter. We never discussed attractions between villagers and volunteers, but they were there, below the surface, creating just enough waves to be noticeable. I remembered how I dreaded and anticipated Carl's return to the clinic after he had left me in charge, how the patients and their problems wore me down day after day.

When Rick turned and left the office, I found myself staring out the window instead of preparing my lecture. I was thinking again about Mexico, about being in charge when Carl was gone. There were the weird cases that I had to look up in books—people who came from hundreds of miles away with incurable diseases—and there were the cases involving people I knew who weren't sure whether they could trust me to make the right decision. And in either situation, I felt responsible, unworthy, but I was all that they had. Strangely, years later, I still felt that way when I had the hopeless cases like Clayton Jones with his sickle-cell anemia.

Chapter Twelve

EVERY DAY, DEANNA'S BROTHER GOYO WOULD CARRY WATER from the river to the clinic to fill our containers. We used a lot of water to clean our tables and supplies and to give to the thirsty patients in the waiting room. Goyo concentrated as he filled the dark ceramic pot with water. He took pride in his work, which included this daily trip to the clinic with cool water collected from shallow pools along the riverbank. He made the trip with his donkey, and people often joked that it was the donkey that was the brains of the team. They even looked alike, the donkey swaybacked and dusty and Goyo hunched over, sand and dust on his face, with his tongue protruding from his thick round lips, which he smacked and licked as he carried water from house to house. His ears stuck out low on his face like two huge plates, all the more noticeable because of his balding head. People called out to him as he walked, but he did not stop to shake hands or talk, preferring to wave his hand in a vibrating upward motion while continuing on with his task. It was as if any disturbance, no matter how small, might permanently alter his path, and he would be forever lost. "That's how he's always been," Deanna told me. One day, after he brought our water, I thanked him, and he nodded as he trudged back to the donkey. As he left, a woman and her baby walked into the room. She looked around at the shelves of medicines and down at the dirt floor. Shaking the dust off her blue silk dress, she averted her eyes as she greeted me. I smiled and waited for her to begin, to tell me the problem.

Sometimes, like that day, it took a half hour for the whole story to come out. "My baby can't walk."

I examined the baby's feet: no signs of any injury or infection. I examined his hips and knees. They moved normally as I bent and turned them.

"How long?" I asked. "When did he begin to have trouble walking?"

"Today. He can't walk today."

"Oh, it just started today?"

"Yes, and yesterday."

I looked in the books for an explanation. The possibilities ranged from bone problems to neurologic diseases to tumors to infections of the spine.

I examined the spine and found a surgical scar.

"What's this?" I asked.

"It's his surgery."

"For what?"

"He was born with it. A hole in his spine." Now the woman looked down, avoiding my eyes. Her secret, her baby's secret revealed. She had long black hair braided down her back; her clothes suggested another place, a city, far from this mountain village.

"Oh, so he has never walked," I said.

"No," she said. "The doctors who operated on him told me that nothing could be done, that he will never walk. But I heard about this clinic. A woman who was blind came here, and now she can see. So I had to try . . . for him. Please, can you help?"

I read the chapters on my likely diagnoses—spina bifida and meningomyelocele. She had medical records from Mexico City. I read them and realized that specialists had already explained the condition and the prognosis. I had nothing further to add.

"How long did it take you to get here?" I asked.

"Four days," she said.

"I'm sorry. We have no medicine that can cure him. And I'm not really a doctor. I'm just a student."

"But you're an American."

"Yes."

"But I heard that this American clinic has American medicines that are stronger than our Mexican medicines. And American doctors who can do operations."

"I'm sorry," I said. "I can't do operations."

She scooped up her child. I could feel the anger and despair in her look, as if she did not believe me but knew that I would not help and make her son walk.

Then her friend came in. They had traveled together by bus. She brought her son, a boy with a moustache and deep voice. They were an odd pair, this child inside a man's body and his mother, exhausted and frightened, transported from a town hundreds of miles away to finally arrive at their destination only to find me and my little room of medicines. The woman had a long face and dark purple lipstick that accentuated her thin lips. Her eyebrows had been plucked bare. She smoked as she explained to me how she and her friend had decided to come here with their children.

"We go to the same clinic together, on the bus," she said, "so we came here together."

"How old is your son?" I asked. He looked to be about the size of an eight- or nine-year-old child.

"He's five years old," she said.

I examined him: his face and neck, his heart, lungs, stomach, genitals. The genitals were fully mature with pubic hair. I called Luis over and showed him.

"If he's this big now, he'll be like a donkey when he's grown up," he said.

"No, Luis, it's some kind of disease or hormone problem. It's not funny," I said. But Luis was laughing as they stood there, the boy exposed, staring up at his mother.

"He's so embarrassed," she said. "Can he put his pants back on?"

"Yes," I said.

Then she showed me medical records from a hospital. His illness was some kind of rare anemia. And the treatment was testosterone, the male hormone. She had the medication with her. That explained the premature puberty, the sexual maturation. I looked it up in my books and found the anemia. The boy's treatment was exactly what my book recommended. I showed the woman my book, and she nodded.

"I'm sorry; there's nothing else I can do for him," I said.

She took three quick puffs from her cigarette and then extinguished it on her chair and dropped it onto the floor.

"Is it true," she asked, "that a woman must not look at the moon when she is pregnant?"

"Well," I said, "I haven't heard that."

"It is a belief we have. If a woman looks at the moon when she is pregnant, her baby will be damaged."

"It is a superstition. The moon cannot affect a baby," I said.

She paused and lit a cigarette. "I looked at the moon," she said. "I was in a cornfield after his conception, and I looked at the moon for an hour and imagined the moon inside of me. And that's why this happened to him."

"No, I don't think so," I said.

"And my friend. She did it also. She fell asleep on a hammock and woke up and looked at the moon before she realized what she had done."

"But you have these reports," I said. "They explain the problem, and there is nothing about the moon. Sometimes things like this just happen."

"No, it is the will of God. I pray to the Virgin every day, and she talks to me. She told me to come here, that you Americans would help us."

"Sometimes American doctors visit the clinic, and usually Dr. Wilson is here. But he had to leave for a while. Perhaps you could come back when he is here."

I didn't really believe in miracles. But there were events and coincidences that defied explanation: people who survived fatal wounds, animals that returned home after traveling hundreds or thousands of miles, a farmer who found a diamond under a kernel of corn. Were they just mathematical oddities, like winning the lottery? If enough time passed, even the most unlikely event would eventually happen. Or was there a pattern—confusing, vague perhaps, but a pattern nonetheless—that needed to be deciphered before the reason for the event could become clear? A cause and an effect, the moonlight and an abnormal baby. And if that was the cause, could there be a cure?

So many times over the years, I've sat in the trauma room with the parents of a dying child hit by a car and searched for some explanation of negligence, alcoholism, or hyperactivity. But often there is no explanation, and what happened is not fair. The suffering is not fair. Why this child? Why these parents? And there's nothing to be done but be there with them.

I imagined the long bus trip over potholes at night, the bus-station food, and the uncertainty about connections and sleep. The moonlight that would accompany them would be a constant reminder and explanation for the illness.

Later that day, I watched them depart in the bed of a converted truck equipped with wooden benches for passengers. It would be an uncomfortable trip back for them. They had purchased tortillas and cookies from a tienda and received water from Goyo and his mule. Goyo had barely taken notice of them as he ladled out a drink from a split gourd. And I wondered again about Goyo and how he had turned out this way, and if he could have been different if treated with a hormone or medicine. Luis and I watched from the clinic window, and I knew I would feel relief when they were gone.

"Luis," I said. "Goyo and Deanna are brother and sister. Deanna is smart and beautiful and Goyo is . . ." I hesitated.

"Stupid and ugly," he answered and laughed.

"Well, yes," I said. "Why do you think they are so different?"

He shrugged. "People say that her mother looked at the moon when she was pregnant with Goyo."

Chapter Thirteen

THE MEMORY OF THAT DAY IN THE CLINIC MERGED WITH my memory of the next day, and what I had had to do.

It started the next morning as I sat in Rosa's kitchen waiting for breakfast.

Sopa vieja splattered in the cooking grease as I drank a cup of warm milk flavored with powdered coffee. Rosa cooked the leftover tortillas with egg and tomato for my breakfast while she directed her children to help with various tasks.

"Tomás, take this to your father for lunch," she would yell, handing a few rolled-up tortillas with beans to the eager eleven-year-old. And off he would go on muleback, riding miles into the mountains where Ricardo tended cattle. Or she would direct the next oldest, Paulo. "Run and get some eggs from the chickens."

She usually fed me long after Ricardo had gone out to the mountain pastures, even though I was up and at the table by seven o'clock in the morning. I looked forward to this time with Rosa, when we could talk about families or recent cases in the clinic or just sip coffee together.

But on this morning, Ricardo was still at home, and he sat at the table sipping coffee as I ate. He waited until I had finished before asking me, "David, do you mind visiting my father?"

"No, I'd be happy to see him," I said. I had met Ricardo's father, Daniel, a few times. I remembered his firm handshake and how he spoke in almost unintelligible, idiomatic Spanish, smiling as if we shared a great joke. Daniel was the *patrón* of the family, the one who had settled the land and raised the family when Indians still roamed the area. It seemed as if half the village was related to him by blood or through baptism.

"It's his hand," Ricardo said.

There were five of Daniel's adult children around him when I walked in the door of his house, and they all looked up at me. Daniel had drool hanging from his lip, which his oldest daughter wiped with a red cloth.

"What happened?" I asked.

"He woke up this way," Ricardo said. "He cannot talk. He cannot move his right arm."

I grasped the right hand hoping for his energetic handshake, and it fell away limp. His words became a sound. "Mmmmmm," he said as his children strained to understand. "Mmmmmm," he said again.

I decided to examine him and sent Ricardo to the clinic to get my stethoscope and a blood pressure cuff.

"Can he have water or tea? We have a native herb tea," said one of the daughters. I looked at the gray liquid in the cup and smelled the minty, pungent fumes.

"Yes, if he can swallow," I said, noting the steady dripping of saliva from his lip. He drank the tea eagerly but coughed as he swallowed.

"This tea can cure sadness," said another daughter.

"Is he sad?" I asked.

"Yes," she said. "He misses his wife, our mother. She died last year. He wants to be with her; that's why this happened."

"I don't know," I said. "But I think we better give him intravenous fluid instead of letting him drink. I don't think he's swallowing too well. I can put a needle in his vein, and then we just have to watch the bottle and change it when it's empty."

Daniel coughed again, spitting up the tea that had pooled in his mouth—as if to emphasize what I had said. When Ricardo returned, I had the family help me undress Daniel. Even at seventy, Daniel's muscles felt taut, like woven rope fibers. With his strong left arm, he strained to help us remove his shirt.

I listened to his lungs with my stethoscope on his back.

"*Respire*," I said, and he took a breath. Even if he could not talk, he seemed to understand me. The sound in his lungs should have been like air rushing through a straw, but instead it sounded like slurping the last few drops of milk from the bottom of a cup—that bubbly, harsh sound of fluid mixed with air in the straw.

Then I listened to his heart. "*Fuerte*," I said. "It is strong."

"He has always had a strong heart," said Ricardo. "Even when a mountain lion jumped on him, he did not get scared."

Ricardo showed me the scars on his father's back where the mountain lion had scratched him. All of the children admired the scars and ran their fingers over his back. And I wondered why I hadn't noticed them before.

I felt his stomach, which bulged slightly and retreated softly and easily under my hand's pressure.

"He only eats tortillas and beans," Ricardo said. "We bring him chicken or beef, but he won't eat it, ever since my mother died."

His legs were like his arms, only heavier. The left moved, resisting me when I pushed it. The right lay heavy and dead, immobile as I pinched and squeezed.

"He could walk for two days up the mountains without resting," Ricardo said. "Even when he was sixty years old, he could walk to Chilar over ten miles away."

I nodded and told them I would be back with the intravenous fluid and the needle. As I was about to leave, one of the daughters took me aside. "It's a stroke, isn't it?" she asked. "There's no cure for a stroke. He will always be like this."

"I'm not sure," I said. "I have to check in the books. Maybe there are some medicines . . ."

She smiled at me as I walked back to the clinic.

The waiting room at the clinic was almost full. A woman sitting on the floor blocked the door to the room where we kept supplies, and I had to watch her show me her child's rash before she would move. "Momentito," I lied. "I'll be back in just a moment." I gathered the plastic tubing, glass bottle of sugar and salt solution, needle, tape, and connecting pieces. By the time I returned to Daniel's house, something had changed. He lay there with his eyes closed, breathing rapidly.

"What happened?" I asked.

"He had a seizure. His whole body shook, even his arms and legs. And then he just fell asleep," said Ricardo.

"It was the tea," said Ricardo's sister. "The herbs have to clean his body like this—remove the sadness—but maybe it was too strong for him."

"What kind of herbs were they?"

"Just a native herb that we call black apple of the devil."

After that, he fell into a deep coma. His breaths would accelerate as if he were having a nightmare and then stop as if he were dead. The family's cries alternated with the rhythm of his breathing. A sob, a brief pause, and then the breaths would start again, slow at first, then faster, speeding out of control, and then nothing.

They sent for a doctor from the city, and he came in an old Chevy. Sometimes, when the road was dry, a car could complete the trip in four hours. Other times, the arroyos filled with water, making the road impassible. They were lucky on this day, as the doctor arrived after hours of bouncing over boulders. He wore a white shirt hanging out of blue polyester pants, and a green and white plaid tie. He sweated and farted as he circled the room, observing the intravenous fluid, the gasping of Daniel, and the single bed in the corner of the room. Finally he wrote a prescription for antibiotics and agreed that the case was hopeless unless God would perform a miracle. He recommended that we all pray. Then he collected his fee and disappeared.

"He said you were doing everything right," said Ricardo. "We trusted you, but my sisters wanted to call him. He is a famous doctor in the city. We had to do it for our father."

"I understand," I said. But I realized that this doctor from the city knew nothing about Daniel. And he never would. The doctor would remember the stench of the room and the dirty blankets, the dust on the road, the heat that made sweat drip from his forehead, and the fee that he collected, stuffed into his hand by Ricardo, who suddenly looked uncertain and small as he said his thank-yous.

In the night, Daniel began to burn with fever. We sat by lantern light and watched as he struggled to breathe.

"He's a fighter," said Ricardo. "He will not give up." Every time the breathing stopped, I hoped it was finally over. And every time, it started again.

"Does he know we are here?" Ricardo whispered.

"Yes," I said. "I think so."

Finally, as the roosters were beginning to crow just before the first light, he died. That last breath came as a shudder. Ricardo said, "*Ya.*" That's it. And we waited until we were sure. And then everyone cried.

"He was so strong, he wouldn't die," said Ricardo as we walked back to the house. "But finally my mother called him to her, and he came." I realized that even though I had spent the entire night awake at the bedside, I was not tired. I felt energized, alive, and I understood how much I had changed since that first night with the baby, that I could feel like I was doing something useful by just being there with them, so that when death arrived they were not alone.

We ate sopa vieja for breakfast, and Tomás brought us warm milk fresh from the cow.

"*Gracias, mi hijo,*" said Ricardo as he hugged his son in a long awkward embrace that wouldn't end. "He's my son," Ricardo said as tears appeared under his eyes, and he continued to squeeze Tomás. I watched the coils of smoke from the fire rise past them as Ricardo leaned from his chair and Tomás stood stiffly staring at the wall. "My son," he said again.

"Yes," I said, as he finally released the boy.

Chapter Fourteen

THE PHONE RANG, SNAPPING ME OUT OF MY REVERIE. I LOOKED at my watch as I answered and realized the residents were already waiting for me.

"Hello," I said.

"This is Max from security."

"Oh, hi, Max. Don't we have a meeting later?"

"Yeah, but this can't wait," he said.

"What is it?" I asked.

"One of your students. He's parking in Mr. T's spot."

"Are you sure?" I asked.

"Oh, yes, we have it on videotape," he said.

I was surprised because Mr. T, a longtime university administrator, had a very recognizable parking space. And we all knew his car, the blue BMW. It would be foolhardy to park in his space. "Who is it?" I asked. "Which resident?"

"The name is Goodman," he said.

"Nancy Goodman?" I asked. "That's hard to believe. I've never had any trouble with her. She always shows up on time."

"Probably because she's parking in Mr. T's spot. He's pretty angry. Wants me to tow the car."

"Is she parked there now?"

"Right now as we speak. That's why I'm calling you now."

"Well, I will talk to her immediately. This will not happen again," I said.

I walked into the room where the residents and students were waiting. Among them was Nancy Goodman. She was from New York and had short, dark hair and a round, happy face perched upon a muscular body. She liked to rock climb and mountain bike. Everyone liked her because she laughed easily, even in life-and-death situations, and liked to make off-color sexual jokes.

"Nancy," I said, "I just got a call from security. Your car . . ." I paused, waiting for her to interrupt and acknowledge her error, explain, and run out to her car. But she waited silently. "Your car is parked illegally. It's about to be towed. It's in Mr. T's spot."

"Oh, he told me I could park there," she said.

"He did?" I asked.

"Oh, yes, he did," she said.

"Well, security doesn't know anything about it. They are about to tow you. You better hurry down there and try to explain. Why would Mr. T let you park there in his space?" I asked.

"We've become friends," she said.

"What? Mr. T? Friends?"

Nancy Goodman smiled as if to answer my incomplete thought.

"OK, well, I don't want to know any more about this. We need to talk privately. You better do something, or your car is going to be towed. You can't reason with security. They just follow the rules. Most of us believe that it is unfair that administrators have special parking spaces and doctors don't. But that's not going to change today. You better move your car until we can sort this out. And I need to begin my lecture on malpractice."

"I'll talk to Mr. T. He'll take care of it," she said and walked out of the conference room.

"Wow," I said. "I can't believe it. How long has this been going on?" I asked the other residents and students.

They looked back at me and shrugged. My secretary came into the room. "There's a telephone call for you," she said. "Mr. T needs to talk to you."

"I'll take it in my office," I said.

"Take a fifteen-minute break," I told the residents. "We'll start after the break."

I picked up my phone. "Hello?" I said.

"It's Mick," he said.

"Oh, hi, Mr. Tomasan," I said. I had never called him Mick, nor even heard anyone call him by his first name.

"Well, I just wanted to let you know that I gave Nancy Goodman approval to park in the administrative area for today," he said.

"You did?" I asked.

"Yes," he said.

"Oh," I said. "So her car?"

"It's been taken care of."

"Oh, so she doesn't have to move it?"

"No."

"Because security called," I said.

"It's not a problem," he said. "She'll be up in just a few minutes."

"It's OK. We're taking a break. Fifteen minutes."

"Excellent," he said. "I'll let her know."

"Good-bye," I said and hung up the phone.

I stood there in shock. I had not seen it coming at all. Nancy had never seemed like anyone who would be involved in a relationship with Mr. T. And Mr. T had always seemed so much older, so conservative, religious—a rock. Perhaps it was a temporary infatuation or just a flirtation, something to break the boredom. I wondered what I'd say when I saw him, what we'd be thinking.

This new secret about a suddenly revealed relationship reminded me of the days before Carl returned to Mexico, when I was carrying around *his* secret. Perhaps there were many secret relationships going on all the time, but I didn't want to know about them. They raised too many questions about how people treat each other. And I could spend hours thinking about them when I was trying to get to sleep.

Back then, I was so worried about getting awakened for an emergency, that I hardly slept at night. I had nightmares about my patients, about the músico or the woman with tetanus. Unlike the thousands of patients who have passed through my emergency department since then, these were people I knew, whose homes I had visited, whose families continued to visit me. Each of them had a story, and I had played a role in the story. Even now, almost thirty years later, I can still see their faces and feel the fear: the man with the huge goiter in his neck hidden under a scarf; the woman with a fungus eating away her scalp. Sometimes when something goes wrong, I remember those first patients, and how alone I was. I had already watched three people die, and I didn't want to watch any more.

Tony's tale continued to echo in my mind, and I wondered how I would react after Carl's return—when we were alone, or when I saw him with Luis. Would I say anything? Would I pretend it was an innocent friendship like everyone else did? Or would I accept it as Luis had?

But then Demetrio arrived.

He came on a stretcher of pine saplings and blankets, carried by four men. They dripped with sweat and mud from carrying him for miles over river crossings and horse trails.

"What happened?" I asked.

They looked at each other, seeking a spokesperson. "A burn," said one man in a straw cowboy hat, and then he looked down at the floor.

"A burn?" I asked as I came closer to the stretcher.

"Yes."

The stretcher was an impressive piece of workmanship: two long posts still covered with bark and lashed together with two smaller posts. Woven blankets stretched over the poles. The man on the stretcher looked up at me with anxious eyes that darted about the room as he grimaced in pain. His legs were exposed, and huge blisters of skin ballooned out like plastic bags filled with air. Around the blisters, discolored splotches of red, gray, and pink skin indicated different severities of burns. He writhed around on the stretcher, and I noticed his arms also had blisters and splotches.

"¡Ay, Dios!" he screamed.

One of the men who had carried him asked, "Don't you have some medicine for him, for the pain?"

"Yes, yes," I said. "Let's move him to bed." By this time a crowd had arrived to find out what was going on. Deanna, Luis, and Tony appeared, accompanied by people from the street, neighbors, shop owners, Ricardo, Tomás, and the man who owned the little store where we bought our Cokes and Fantas.

"Luis," I said, "could you get me the intravenous fluid and the needles and tubing, and then we can give him some pain medicine."

I excused myself and hurried into our consultation room with all my books and began to read about burns. Burns were classified into three degrees of severity. First-degree burns were the least severe and could be recognized by the redness and pain of the skin, but there was no blistering. It was like a bad sunburn. A second-degree burn was more serious and involved blisters with red, tender skin underneath and on the edges. Because nerve endings were exposed and alive in the second-degree burns, these were very painful, but the burns usually healed without the need for skin grafting, as long as they did not become infected. Third-degree burns were the most severe. They were deep burns that killed the nerves and the skin cells, and because of that, they were not painful. They could be gray or white or even black and generally would not heal without a skin graft. The amount of burned surface was also important because the greater the surface involved, the more fluid could be lost, increasing the need for replacement fluid. Some burn victims needed gallons of fluid every day to replace what they were losing. The most feared complications of burns were infections of the burned skin and burn damage to the lungs from inhalation of smoke. The book recommended transferring patients with burns over more than 10 percent of their body surface to a specialized hospital for burns. The diagram in the book showed that each leg was 18 percent of the total body surface. And each arm was 9 percent. I estimated that my patient had 20–30 percent of his body surface area involved.

I returned to the room to find him on a bed. From what I could see, most of the burns were first and second degree. The left arm had a few blisters. The right arm had some redness but no blisters. His face was sweaty but not burned, and he was not coughing. I listened with my stethoscope; his lungs sounded clear.

"Here is the intravenous catheter," said Luis.

He handed me a needle inside a plastic sheath. I had to stick this into a vein and then tape it in place and connect it with tubing to the bottle of intravenous fluid. I selected the arm without blisters and cleaned an area over a vein with an alcohol swab. I had watched the placement of intravenous catheters several times and had put in a few, but never for a burn patient. I made sure to avoid any areas of redness and stuck the needle through the skin. The vein was large and easy to feel and see. As the needle entered the vein, blood appeared at the end of the catheter; I slid the catheter over the needle and pulled the needle out. Blood dripped out of the end of the catheter onto the floor.

"OK, I got it," I said.

We taped the catheter in place and connected the tubing and the intravenous fluid. I watched the steady display of drops as the fluid entered the vein.

Then I injected morphine into the intravenous line in small amounts, the way the book recommended, until the pain began to diminish.

"What is your name?" I asked the young man as he became more able to communicate.

"Demetrio," he said.

"What happened?"

"It was a fire. We were cooking, and I had a can of kerosene for the lantern, and it exploded and I got burned," he said.

"You have pretty bad burns. You should go to a special hospital in town that has specialists in burn care, because the burns can become infected," I said.

I looked at his face, and I could see past the pain that had been contorting him. He had a round face with big cheeks that tried to form a smile when he relaxed. He looked down and did not answer.

"How does that sound?" I asked.

"Well, it's just that I don't want to go to the hospital," he said. "I feel better now."

"Yes, well, that is because of the pain medicine. But it will wear off. And we have to clean your burns and put on medicine. It will take days, maybe weeks, for this to heal, and we are only a little clinic," I said.

He nodded. "Gracias," he said.

I called Deanna, Luis, and Tony together to discuss what we should do.

"I could take him in my truck," said Tony.

"I don't think he wants to go," I said. "We could clean the burns and keep him here until tomorrow when Carl gets back."

"I think maybe this man was not telling us the true story," said Luis. "His friends are talking about soldiers who might come here. They are afraid and want to go."

"Why would soldiers come here?" I asked.

"Maybe drugs. Maybe he was growing some marijuana or opium."

"Opium?" I asked. "Does opium grow here? I've heard about marijuana but not opium."

"Yes," said Luis. "Opium and marijuana."

"They're all pigs," said Tony. "The police, the soldiers. What's wrong with a little dope?"

"I think we should clean the burns and let him stay here. Come on, Antonio, you can help me," said Deanna, and she went to find bandages, ointment, and forceps to clean and treat the burns.

"Demetrio," I asked, "why don't you want to go to the hospital? They will have better treatments for your burn."

Demetrio looked at his friends. Their eyes met wordlessly and lingered for a few seconds. Then he looked away and back at me. He smiled. "Thank you for your treatment. I can go back to my home now with my friends."

"No, that is not necessary. We can keep you here for a while. We can remove some of the dead skin, apply some ointment to your burns, and give you fluid in your vein. Tomorrow Dr. Wilson will return, and he can decide what we should do. You can stay here in the clinic in that bed. Your friends can bring you food."

"I can pay you," he said, and he pulled out a roll of ten- and twenty-dollar bills.

Luis whistled.

"No, no, it's free here. Later, if you would like to give a donation to the clinic, we would be grateful. But you may need your money for food and drinks."

"Thank you," he said. "When my nephew was here, you treated him and now he is fine," he said.

"What nephew?" I asked.

"A small baby," he said. "You touched his head and stopped his seizure."

"I, well, a seizure can just stop. It was my first day. I don't remember you. Just the mother and father."

"He was my brother. I helped dig the hole in the ground for the latrine. Don't you remember?" he said.

But the first days were still a blur to me. I remembered blisters on my hands and sleeping in Ricardo's house. Now Ricardo came over to me. "This boy is my godson," he said. "How serious is it?"

"He should be in a hospital with a burn specialist," I said.

"Very well," he said. "I will make the arrangement to take him there."

"Well, he does not want to go," I said.

Ricardo conversed quietly with Demetrio. They argued and nodded and spoke too quickly for me to understand it all. Finally, Ricardo said, "This boy is very stubborn. He will not go to the hospital. Is it possible to treat him here?"

"Yes, we can try," I said. "Is his father or family coming?"

The boy looked at me and then explained to Ricardo that his father was up in the high mountains with the cattle. There were soldiers who would steal the cattle if someone was not watching. That was why the other friends would have to go back.

"No," said Ricardo, "his father cannot come here. I will be responsible for him."

"He will need to drink a lot of fluids and eat good food."

"Hot or cold?" said Ricardo.

"Well, I don't think it matters. Juices, soup, Cokes."

"Very well," said Ricardo. "*Con permiso.*" He nodded and turned and left.

Deanna and Tony helped me remove the broken blisters from Demetrio's legs. The skin came off in delicate sheets like tissue paper, and it shriveled up into tiny balls as it lay drying on a plastic tray. As the damaged skin came off, smooth, pink, glistening new skin appeared.

"We need to clean and scrub the skin," I said. But as we rubbed the new pink skin with sterile antibiotic solution and brushes, Demetrio cried out in pain. Even more morphine could not make the pain endurable. So we rinsed the skin with water and applied antibiotic ointment and covered it all with antibiotic bandages.

To pass the time and distract him, I asked Demetrio questions.

"How old are you?"

"Eighteen."

"Do you go to school?"

"I went to the first grades. But I had to live here in town, and I missed my family too much, so I stopped," he said.

"You stopped," I said.

"Yes, I had to help my father with the cattle. I miss the girls," he said.

"Girls?"

He grinned widely for the first time. "We don't have many girls in the mountains."

"Just *burras*, goats, and sheep," Luis said, laughing, and he slapped his hand to Demetrio's.

"*¡Ay, Dios!*" yelled Demetrio as a piece of skin was pulled from his leg.

"*Lo siento*," I said. Sorry. "How did the fire start?"

"I don't know exactly. I was holding a bottle of kerosene, pouring it into one of our lanterns, and it just exploded. Maybe it was from lightning."

"Lightning?" I asked.

"Sometimes lightning can do this," he said.

"Did you put any medicine on your burns?" I asked.

"Only herbs. My mother put some herbs on my legs, but they fell off when we were crossing the river," he said.

"Well, now, we will put on medicine, and we will have to cover it with bandages and change the bandages every day. It could take days or weeks before the burns heal."

"So, I will stay here?" he asked.

"Yes, well, until Dr. Wilson returns. Then we will discuss it with him."

Carl returned in the middle of the night. I heard the motor of the Jeep idling outside the clinic and jumped out of bed to greet him. I tried to focus on how I would report the events of the past week—the deaths, the clinic visits, this new burn patient—and not talk about what Tony had shared or reveal that I was upset and confused about it. Luis was already there, grabbing boxes and suitcases and bringing them into the clinic. I joined him in unloading the Jeep. Carl nodded at me. "Here, take these boxes," he said and handed me large cardboard boxes filled with donated medicines.

"Carl, I need to tell you about a burn patient who is in the clinic," I said.

"Yes, I already saw him. Luis told me about him. He needs to be in a hospital burn unit."

"I know. But he doesn't want to go to a burn unit."

"Let's discuss it in the morning. I've been driving for twenty hours straight. I need to get some sleep."

It was not the conversation I had expected—or practiced. I had imagined we would discuss my patients, and he would thank me for doing my best. And then, I had thought, we would weigh the options for Demetrio and make a plan together. And finally, we would talk about Luis and Tony and the others and how uncomfortable it made me feel. Instead, I unpacked boxes and piled them in the clinic as Carl disappeared into the loft. I was left alone listening to the sounds of the street and Demetrio snoring in the back of the clinic.

When I woke up the next day, a military Jeep was parked outside the clinic next to Carl's Jeep. Gabriel was at the clinic door. "*Federales*," he said in a whisper.

Inside the clinic, three soldiers in camouflage battle fatigues were talking with Carl. One soldier had glasses, a moustache, and cap, and seemed a bit older than the other two, who looked no more than seventeen.

"He is under arrest for violation of drug laws," said the soldier with glasses.

"He has very serious burns," said Carl. "He cannot be moved."

The soldiers carried rifles. They walked into the room where Demetrio lay, looked at the bandages on his legs, and returned to the front of the clinic.

"We will return tomorrow," said the soldier with the glasses. "He must remain here."

"Of course," said Carl. "He can't even walk, so he will not be going anywhere else."

The soldier nodded and motioned to the other two to follow him. They jumped onto their Jeep and sped off in a cloud of dust.

"What happened?" I asked.

"Oh, our burn patient seems to be in a bit of difficulty," said Carl. "The federales believe he was involved in processing opium into heroin when he caught on fire. They want to take him to prison."

"What should we do?" I asked.

"If we let them take him, he will probably die in jail of his burns, or they will just shoot him and throw him in a ditch. We've seen that here before. But if we keep him here, they will keep coming back and causing problems. And anyway, I don't want to protect drug producers. Drugs are ruining the village."

"Maybe he didn't do it. He said it was a kerosene lamp that blew up."

"Well, that's also possible, but we won't be able to convince the soldiers of that."

Luis walked into the room.

"Hi, Luis," I said.

"Hola, David."

"Did you see the soldiers?" I asked.

"*Sí*, it is what I told you yesterday."

"Well, who knows?" I said.

"We have saved him for today, but he is endangering the clinic and everything we have built over years, and we cannot risk it," said Carl. "We are going to have to make some difficult decisions."

"Shouldn't we at least include Demetrio in the decision, since it's about him?" I asked.

Carl paused for a moment, considering my suggestion. He turned and smiled at me. "I suppose you are right. After all, we are trying to involve the people who are affected by the diseases, to have them participate in curing themselves. That is our philosophy, the empowerment of the poor. This would be a good example of the philosophy, and if it is correct, Demetrio will participate in his own solution."

I nodded without fully comprehending Carl's response. But at least I could see that he had accepted my suggestion.

I followed him into the room where Demetrio lay under a sheet. Carl sat on the cot and picked up the sheet, exposing Demetrio's legs and the bandages covering the burns.

"Well, young man," he said, "how are you feeling today?"

"Good," said Demetrio.

"Those burns will take quite some time to heal, probably weeks. We cannot keep you here for weeks."

Demetrio looked down at the floor. "I am very grateful for all of the treatment you have given me. I feel much better now. My legs feel better. I think I can ride a horse back to our place."

"You know there were soldiers here this morning. They have some questions. We told them you would not leave until they can talk to you."

"Yes," said Demetrio.

Carl put his hand on Demetrio's thigh and rubbed it gently up and down a few times. "I don't feel any sign of infection," said Carl.

"Thank you," said Demetrio.

"But I think you should stay here for a few more days. I will talk to the soldiers."

Demetrio nodded.

"Well, he's young and fit. A few days of treatment here, and then perhaps the soldiers can take him in for a visit. But they may be off on another hunt by then. You did a nice job in the burn debridement."

"Thanks," I said. "It's been a difficult week and a half."

"Yes, three deaths. That's a lot for this village."

"So, you heard about them?"

"Yes, Luis told me about them. It's shocking that in this day we are still seeing deaths from tetanus. Our vaccination program must reach all of the people, not just the children. And of course, the death of Ricardo's father is a terrible loss for all of us. But, you know, people here do not survive long with strokes or any disability. There is no support for them, no nursing care. So they tend to die. No lingering for weeks or months or years like in the United States."

"I never realized people would be dying here," I said. "I thought we would treat them, and they would either get better or, if they were very sick, go to a hospital. But they don't want to go to the hospital."

"No, they do not believe that hospitals are places to get better. They trust God and they trust us. And if they go to the hospital, they have to find money to pay for the X rays and medicine."

"So what will we do with Demetrio?"

"I will try to delay things. I think we need time to give this situation a chance to become clear."

I nodded. Carl turned and walked toward the clinic door. "I'll be back in an hour. I need to meet with the mayor and find out more about the soldiers. You can open the clinic as you have been doing."

"OK," I said. As I headed over to see Demetrio, I realized that I had not talked to Carl about Luis or the story that Tony had told me. Carl's statement about a delay to let the situation with the federales become clear seemed reasonable. Demetrio looked up from his cot. I noticed he had a small plate of beans and tortillas. He was dipping his tortillas into the beans and then chewing on the tortillas.

"Hi, Demetrio," I said. "Someone got you food."

"Yes, my girlfriend, Carmen, is here," he said. He pointed to a figure sitting quietly in the corner. The figure raised her head in acknowledgment before reassuming her previous pose. I could not see her eyes. She wore a tan skirt and white blouse, and a red and green woven shawl covered her head, neck, and shoulders. Long black hair in braids trailed down her back. Her dark brown skin was smooth and clear except for a mole on her chin.

"I didn't know you had a girlfriend," I said. He smiled and lifted his eyebrows as if he had shared some intimate secret with me.

"She's my girlfriend, and we plan to marry," he said.

"Well, congratulations," I said. "We have been discussing your situation. Carl has decided to let you stay here for a few days, and then you will have to go with the soldiers to clear up this problem. We are hoping that a few days of treatment will be enough to prevent the infection."

"Very good," said Demetrio. "I am trying to drink lots of juices and Cokes. Look at all the bottles." And he showed me a collection of Coke bottles and empty juice tins. "I feel strong."

"Good," I said. I felt his forehead. "You don't have a fever, so everything is going well. Now I have to see other patients in the clinic. Deanna and Tony will be by later to see if you need to have any more blisters removed."

"Thank you," he said.

I returned to the consultation room. The waiting room was full, and the first patient who limped into my consultation room was an old man with an infected toe. It had been going on for two weeks. I examined it, cleaned away the pus, and gave him a plastic bag with antibiotics. By the time Carl returned, I had seen six patients and handed out six bags with medicine, and Gabriel had filled out a card on each patient that listed the name, diagnosis, and treatment.

Carl told me he had discussed the problem of the soldiers with the mayor. The mayor told Carl the soldiers were bad for business in town. They bothered the young girls and scared the merchants. He asked Carl to give him some money to pay off the colonel in charge of the soldiers.

"What?" I said. "That's bribery. Why should we give money to the mayor?"

"That's how things work here," said Carl. "Anyway, I just came back from the foundation, so I have money. But I will wait for a while, and we can see what they do."

In the afternoon I heard some noise in the back and thought Demetrio might need some more morphine for pain. As I went to check on him, I heard the cot creaking, and there was a gentle swaying of bodies—Demetrio and Carmen. They did not notice as I watched. He held her close and stared up at the ceiling as she bent down and kissed his neck. She seemed too small on top of him. Her braids fluttered in the air. I turned quietly and walked out.

The next day the soldiers returned.

Carl explained that Demetrio's burns were not healed. The soldiers walked through the clinic, picking up small bottles of medicine and looking at shelves. They came over to Demetrio and looked at his bandages. They asked him his name and where he lived. Finally, they agreed to return the next day.

That day I worked in the clinic again. Carl went to visit the mayor, and I wondered if he took money with him. I visited Demetrio after lunch. He was laughing and joking with Luis, Carmen, and Tony.

"You seem happy. Why?" I said.

"My friends keep telling me jokes," he said. "They told me that a man walked on the moon."

"It's true," I said.

"It is not possible," he said. "How can you get there?"

"On a rocket ship," I said.

Demetrio began to laugh, looked at Carmen, and then they both burst into laughter. Soon we were all laughing.

That night, Demetrio disappeared. And it was not only Demetrio. Tony, Deanna, and Carmen were also gone. His burns were getting better, but I never expected he would leave. When the soldiers came, we tried to explain.

"He left suddenly in the night," said Carl. "We have no idea where he went."

"Where is he? You must show us where he is," said a soldier.

"No, he's not here. He left in the night," Carl said again.

"He was too sick to escape. Where is he? Where did you put him?"

"No, he left in the night. We are very sorry," said Carl.

When the soldiers realized what had happened, they became confused and searched the clinic, wondering if some language problem had created a false impression. Then they became angry. I could see their faces change color as they began to swear, first at each other, then at us. And then they pointed their guns. I watched Carl as the soldiers screamed at him. He remained calm, treating them the way a high school teacher would treat unruly students, explaining things calmly and ignoring their threats. He didn't seem to feel in danger. Finally, the soldiers began to break things. They tore the clinic apart, breaking bottles of medicines. All of Deanna's sorting and Loli's cleaning and all of the donated medicines and supplies from the United States were destroyed in an hour. We stood by and watched. As we stood at the doorway watching and listening, I said, "It's over. It's destroyed, and when they're done, they'll probably shoot us or arrest us."

"No," said Carl. "They're just boys. This is what boys do. It's a teen-age temper tantrum. They're angry, and when they've broken enough things, they will leave."

"And what about us?"

"They don't want us. We are too much of a complication for them."

"Well, I . . . I don't know if I can stay here."

"You can take the bus tomorrow if you want. But we need you. The people need you even more than ever. We can send you up into the mountains away from the village into the sierra where the true beauty of this place and these people will be clearer. Or you can help me in the clinic or work as a dentist. There's so much you can do now that you understand Spanish and you have learned so much medicine. Look, the patients are already lined up waiting for us, for this to be finished."

I looked around behind me, and there were patients—mothers holding children, a man with a bandanna around his large swollen jaw.

"OK," I said.

We closed the clinic that day and salvaged what we could. Most of the spills had come from relatively few bottles. Carl drove to Durango and bought replacement medicine. By the next day, we were open for business. We knew that Deanna and Tony had also disappeared with Demetrio, but we did not learn exactly what happened until several days later when we received a letter from Tony and Deanna.

Don Carlos, Luis, Loli, David, sorry for the surprise. Demetrio had been planning it with his brothers for days. They were sneaking into the clinic at night and visiting with him. We couldn't let him get caught after all our work on his skin. So we drove him and Carmen to Chamisal Arroyo and his brothers had a horse waiting. Then we drove out past two checkpoints. The soldiers would have found him at the checkpoints. They almost took

Deanna because some of her identification papers were expired. But Deanna talked her way out of it. We've just crossed over into Texas. We're all safe. More later. *Hasta luego, amigos.*

Tony and Deanna

Carl and I looked at each other. We were both surprised, and we were very relieved that everyone was safe.

"Demetrio, his brothers, Tony, and Deanna all planned this," said Carl. "And I even paid the colonel and the mayor."

"Really?" I said. "How much?"

"One hundred dollars," said Carl. "But it's not over. There will be another chapter to this story."

"What do you mean?" I asked.

Carl shook his head and walked away.

Chapter Fifteen

RICK CAME BACK INTO THE OFFICE, INTERRUPTING MY thoughts. "They're waiting for you, all the young doctors, waiting for you to impart the wisdom of why to be a doctor."

"Rick, I don't think I can face them. I just found out that Nancy Goodman may be having an affair with Mr. T," I said.

"Really? With Mr. T?" Rick laughed. "That's great. We'll all be able to get free parking spaces."

"Rick, it's not funny. She's thirty years younger than he is. This is going to be a disaster. We have a responsibility to her."

"It's her life. In Saudi Arabia, Mr. T would be marrying a fifteen-year-old girl. We're only responsible to teach her how to read EKGs, treat asthma, sew people up. Just the doctor stuff, like in *Doctor Kildare*, *Ben Casey*, and *Marcus Welby, M.D.*"

"Nothing like this happened on *Marcus Welby, M.D.* or *Doctor Kildare*," I said.

"Well, those guys never even had to look things up in books. And they only had sex with the wealthy widows of the dead patients. Except Kildare, who was gay," said Rick.

Rick went to my bookshelf and pulled out some old emergency medicine texts. He thumbed through the chapters and started to laugh. "It's all wrong," he said. "All the stuff we told people to do back in the eighties was wrong. We told them to give narcotics for headaches and never get an EKG before taking a history and never give pain medication to people with possible appendicitis. All wrong stuff. So maybe those TV doctors were right to ignore the books." Rick laughed so hard he began coughing.

"Yeah," I said. "We think it's all different now. We think what's in the book is true. It's all supposed to be evidence based."

Rick suddenly slammed the book against the desk, and I jumped. "Why'd you do that?" I asked.

"That's what it's good for—killing flies," he said, and he revealed the crushed fly fragments on the book cover.

"Thanks, Rick," I said.

"You ought to throw them all away. Replace them with travel books and math books."

"Why would I want to do that?" I asked.

"When you get depressed about the ER, if you read a travel book, it's like Prozac. You're not depressed anymore. You start thinking about the weather in Iceland or a festival in Bolivia. It's like reading about all the new stuff in the medical journals that come every week, but you don't have to remember any of it, unless you want to."

"OK, and what about the math books?"

"You need the math books to help your kids with their homework. Really, it's important. You don't want them to think you're stupid. And they never get out-of-date. You never need a new edition. Calculus is still calculus. No one has discovered any new integrals or differentials. But you know kids can't multiply twelve times eight without a calculator. Even the residents can't multiply or divide in their heads. It's becoming a lost art, like weaving or setting type or driving with a clutch. So if you know math, you can make your kids think you're still smart."

"Rick, you're crazy. I'm not going to replace my medical books with travel books and math books. What if a patient had meningitis, and I couldn't remember the antibiotic to use or the dose?"

"Get it online. Everything you need is on a computer. The Web sites update this information every year."

"I don't know. By the time I can find the right site, I've wasted too much time."

"Oh, you are going the way of the dinosaurs," said Rick. "People like you are becoming extinct, like the dodo."

"I know," I said. "We should have become dentists. All you have to know is one thing—teeth. Maybe teeth and gums."

"And they make more money than we do," said Rick. "They don't have to take patients who can't pay, even if their teeth are rotten and falling out. They take Fridays off and never work weekends or nights."

"You know, I used to pull teeth," I said. "Did you know that when I was in Mexico before I went to medical school I pulled teeth?" And before I went into the resident lecture, I told Rick how it had happened.

After the debacle with the soldiers, Carl decided that I should take over the job of the dentist. It was probably good for me to move into the dental room. After practicing medicine alone—making decisions and emergency house calls—I needed to assume a more appropriate support role. Even as I felt relieved, I also missed the importance of my previous activity. But everyone needed a dentist, and though I knew nothing about pulling teeth, I decided I would try it. I had always feared dentists, ever since my own teeth were drilled and filled without anesthetics. Our dentist in Chelsea, Massachusetts, a family friend, did not believe in anesthetics. But he was Jewish, so my parents trusted him. We'd just scream in pain as he drilled; we didn't know any better. It was only when I went away to college that I found out that much of the pain could be blunted with an injection. Still, it was difficult to imagine becoming a dentist and inflicting pain on others. But Luis, who had been doing most of the dental work, was busy helping Carl on a variety of projects. And as the dentist, I could continue to do something helpful. I could become absorbed in the task and not think about the patient, Carl, Luis, Tony, Deanna, or Demetrio. I could be in my own world and still help the clinic. Luis was happy to teach me the techniques of tooth extraction, at which he had become an expert. "It's as easy as kissing an American girl," he'd tell me.

The dental chair was placed in front of a large window with vertical bars. The window was shuttered every evening. In the morning, when the shutters were opened, a small audience often gathered on the other side of the window. Some in the audience were regulars. Doña Mercedes came almost every day to watch. She lived about four houses away and often wore a white dress and a large white hat. Her pale skin and frail eighty-year-old body contrasted with her fierce blue-gray eyes and high-pitched laugh. She and Loli would often cry out together in excitement when a dental extraction was complete.

"*Escupe, escupe!*" Spit, spit. They would yell at the patient, encouraging him to spit up the blood that had pooled in his mouth. Ricardo also loved to watch when he wasn't working. He told me it was like watching a bullfight. He hoped that someday one of his sons might be a dentist.

Other dental patients would sit at the window, watching to find out what was in store for them. The performance convinced some of them that their pain was not so bad, and perhaps they would wait and see if it got better by itself. The people at the window often brought wooden chairs from their homes or from the clinic waiting area for comfortable viewing. A soda vendor sold Coke and Sprite to the audience as the day warmed, and some small-scale wagering often took place concerning how long it would take, whether the patient would stay until completion, or how much blood would be lost.

The dental window was acknowledged to be the best and most consistent entertainment in town, and I was anxious about being in the spotlight. Perhaps if there had been electricity for a light bulb, we could have kept the shutters closed to maintain some privacy. But at that time, it wasn't possible.

Since most of our patients had severely decayed teeth with abscesses, extraction was as much a medical emergency as a procedure for pain relief. Without the extraction, the pus could spread into the sinuses of the face and head and, ultimately, to the brain, causing death. Or it could push up the tongue and block the breathing passage. A person walking the village streets with a large red bandanna covering his face usually had a severely abscessed tooth. The bandanna was placed to hide the obvious swelling, and perhaps sometimes used as a treatment, covering a strong-smelling ointment.

A dental extraction occurred in stages. First, I would inject a local anesthetic, either above the tooth or as a nerve block into the lower jaw. If this was done effectively, it was almost painless and made the tooth numb. A patient who had been in pain would generally get immediate relief from the anesthetic injection and would begin to relax. Without good anesthetic effect, the other steps for tooth extraction were almost impossible. Once the tooth was numb, I would separate the gum from the tooth with a sharp spoon-shaped metal instrument called an elevator. This resulted in moderate bleeding, and the patient might swallow the blood. Next, with an instrument that I called the pliers, I would encircle and grab the tooth. Using a rocking motion, I would loosen the roots, making extraction with a final pull possible. Sometimes, if the roots were particularly deep or crossed, it might take twenty to thirty minutes of rocking the tooth to loosen it sufficiently for extraction. In most cases, once the tooth was removed, there would be bleeding from the socket, and I would stuff cotton balls and gauze into it. If the tooth broke during the extraction, a piece of root might be retained, and I would have to scrape that out with a long sharp instrument. Few physicians know much about dental infections or have ever pulled out a tooth. But over the years, I've learned that variations of this basic approach are still commonly followed among dentists.

Most of my initial patients were desperate to have something done. The pain had been keeping them up for many nights. They had often journeyed for days on muleback over mountain passes to reach the clinic. They felt like they were dying. Once I anesthetized the tooth and the pain eased, they would have allowed me to do anything else I wanted. Luis remained available to help me with difficult cases, and I pulled three or four teeth every day. Some patients asked for extraction of other nondiseased teeth to spare future problems.

One day an elderly man with a red bandanna arrived. Something about his eyes and moustache seemed familiar. Loli brought him to me.

"Don Felipe has a very painful tooth," Loli said. Then he burst into his usual hysterical laughter. "No more music, no more music," he cried.

Then I recognized don Felipe. He was the father of my patient, the músico, who had died.

"Enter, don Felipe." I greeted the old man.

"Ay, dios!" he cried. "Ay, dios!"

I looked in his mouth. There were only four teeth left. They all looked bad, but the one on the lower right was giving him the pain.

"Bueno," I said. "Let's pull it out."

"*Ande le pues*," he muttered. Go ahead.

Before I began, I said, "Don Felipe, if you want someone else to pull your tooth, I could get Luis for you."

"Luis is a little *cabrón*. No, you can do it."

As I was injecting the anesthetic, I noticed that Loli and doña

Mercedes had been joined by some musician friends of don Felipe's son. They sat in chairs, singing and playing guitar. Don Felipe tried to smile at them, but his mouth had a needle in it.

After I separated the gum, I placed the pliers around the tooth. It should have moved easily as I turned my wrist, but it barely budged. I continued to turn my wrist back and forth with maximal effort. The musicians picked up the beat as sweat began to form droplets on my forehead. A fly buzzed around don Felipe's open mouth, and I began praying to myself. "Please don't fly in; please don't fly in." Blood began to pool in the back of his mouth.

"Escupe, escupe!" I said. Spit, spit!

After twenty minutes of constant effort, the tooth was only slightly looser than when I had begun. Don Felipe's eyes gazed up at me plaintively. The anesthetic was beginning to wear off. "Just a few more minutes," I said. I strained against the obstinate tooth. "He can't do it," I heard doña Mercedes whisper to Loli.

After ten more minutes, the tooth was loosening. I could feel it moving. A few more minutes, and I'd have it. With my life defined by the task, the tooth filled my mind, and all I could think about was pulling it out, about not failing.

Then don Felipe raised his hand. His face dripped in sweat as tears flowed from the corners of his eyes. "*No más, ya no más*," he mumbled. No more, no more. He wanted me to stop, just as I was about to pull out the loosened tooth.

"It's ready to come out. I can't stop now. You could swallow it in your sleep."

"No más," he said. "Mañana."

He wanted to return tomorrow. I could hear the murmurs from my audience. "Mañana," they said.

I told don Felipe to wait as I ran to look for Luis. Perhaps Luis could explain and be given the chance to pull it out. I found him in the examining room with Carl.

"Luis," I said. "I have don Felipe in the dental chair. His tooth is almost out, and he wants to leave. Can you come and talk to him?"

Luis came in and looked at the tooth. "It's so loose," he said. "I could pull it out in ten seconds."

But as he explained all this to don Felipe, the old man continued to raise his hand and spit blood.

"Mañana," he repeated.

"He wants to pull it tomorrow," Luis said.

The musicians helped carry him away, down the street, still spitting blood. The image of his dead son's eyes flooded back to me as I watched don Felipe disappear around a corner.

That night as I was sleeping, I began to dream. I heard the mad growls of a rabid dog on the main street next to the clinic. I had heard this fierce growl in my sleep the past two nights and recognized the sound of the fatally infected animal ready to pass the disease to anyone it could bite. The dog terrified and angered me. The randomness of its lethality meant no one was safe. It had to be killed. I would do it with a wooden baseball bat that Ricardo kept in the house for security. I put on my pants and grabbed the bat and a flashlight. Although the dog sounded like it was outside my window, I saw nothing but dirt and shadows when I aimed the light. The dog could be anywhere, lurking in the shadows ready to pounce. I wound the bat back, ready to strike. My heart pounded with an accelerating crescendo as I strained to hear the dog, but the sounds of the dog were gone. Had they ever been there? Then suddenly the dog was snarling, jumping toward my face. I swung at it. And then I woke up sweating. I wondered if I had cried out in terror and awakened the household. But no one seemed to be moving, and I drifted back into a fitful sleep.

The next day, don Felipe was waiting for me. He was ready to have his tooth pulled. I applied the pliers to test how loose it was and realized I could yank it out with one sudden motion. As I suddenly decided and pulled, don Felipe grabbed at his jaw and at my hand. But I had the tooth out. I held it high above my head and then showed it to him. He smiled a bloody smile. Of our audience, only doña Mercedes had arrived to witness the event. I looked at the tooth carefully. The roots were crossed. The enamel was worn down and stained. A cavity covered the inner surface. I gave him the tooth, and he squeezed it into his clenched fist. The socket bled slightly, and I stuffed a cotton ball into it. I was glad to have cured him, but even more, I was glad to be done with it, this demon tooth.

"Come back tomorrow, and I will check it again," I said.

He nodded and opened his fist to show the tooth to doña Mercedes. "*Gracias a Dios,*" she said in her witchlike voice.

As he emerged into the brightness of the day, don Felipe hesitated, allowing his eyes to adjust. A dead dog lay in the street, flies swarming around its bloody mouth.

"Rabies," said doña Mercedes as if answering a question suggested by don Felipe's hesitation at the clinic entrance.

"Yes, rabies," don Felipe said as he walked forward. As he passed the dog, he dropped the rotten tooth that he had been rubbing in his palm and spit bloody saliva into the foamy pool by the dog's mouth.

Chapter Sixteen

"THAT'S WEIRD," SAID RICK. "YOU COULD BE SUED IF YOU pulled teeth in this country."

"Yeah, well you can be sued just about anytime things don't turn out well. And that reminds me, the students and residents are waiting for my malpractice lecture," I said.

"Well, scare them good," said Rick. "I don't want them messing up on my shift." Rick raised his shaggy eyebrows for emphasis, and it reminded me of how he would do that to make a point when we were residents together. In those days there were no faculty to check our work in the hospital at night, and we enjoyed our independence. We never considered the mistakes we might be making or the lawsuits that might follow. Rick would often remind me that the patients were not paying for their care, and in return, they had to have medical students and residents learning medicine on them.

I walked into the lecture room and nodded to the students and residents. I had met some of them a few times, but I still couldn't remember their names, and I was too embarrassed to ask them all to introduce themselves again. There was the blond woman with very light skin and glasses, the tall guy with a beard from the University of Washington, Nancy Goodman from Stony Brook, the older guy from Boston named Matt or Mack, and so on.

"Hi, today's topic is medical malpractice," I said. "I'll be describing the elements of malpractice, the role of experts, what to do if you are named in a suit, the deposition and trial, and impact on your psychological health and subsequent credentialing and privileges. I am going to start with a case.

"A ten-year-old girl came to the emergency department with abdominal pain and diarrhea . . ." I said and described a typical case of appendicitis that was initially misdiagnosed as stomach flu. The girl went home but got worse, and by the time she returned, the appendix had ruptured. I described the physical exam, the laboratory tests, the documentation in the chart, the instructions to the family, and the final outcome.

"Well, how would you know the difference between stomach flu and early appendicitis? They sound almost the same. And we're just interns!" said the blond woman.

"Experience helps," I said. "And not being in a rush or not getting interrupted. But frankly, you are going to miss these sometimes."

"And then you get sued?" she asked.

"Not always," I said. "Actually, lawsuits often come from perfectly fine medical care, when something bad happens that nobody could have anticipated, and then the family needs to find someone to blame. And there's so much money involved. Lawsuits can be worth millions, and the lawyers get a third of that. It's big business. Look at all the ads for malpractice lawyers in the paper."

"Is it like this in other countries?" asked the man with the beard. He squinted and smacked his lips as he talked.

"Like this?" I said. "No, I think we're unique. In other countries, medicine is considered a public service or a public good. Here, it's a business, and no one feels badly about suing a business."

"I'm going to New Zealand when I finish the residency," he said. "They don't have malpractice lawsuits, from what I hear. You may not get rich, but you don't have to worry that every patient will sue you. I think I'd quit medicine if I got sued."

"Yes, several of the doctors I worked with have quit medicine or left the country because of a malpractice suit. Sometimes I get tempted. But if you follow the rules I identified—a good history and physical, appropriate lab, re-examination, documentation, and follow-up— you'll make fewer mistakes, and you'll be less likely to get sued. And listen to the nurses. They will often catch something you might miss. And be careful when you are distracted by personal issues—fights with your spouse, lack of sleep, illness." As I said it, I realized I was a good example of what not to do. When I had worked after learning that my wife was leaving, I could not concentrate on anything. I had no idea what decisions I had made.

We talked some more about the case and about malpractice, and then I concluded the session with stories about Mexico.

As faculty who were getting to know the interns, we were supposed to share something personal. I told them about how I had volunteered in the clinic in Mexico before I started medical school and how I made diagnoses by matching symptoms with diagnoses described in a book called *Differential Diagnosis*.

And I told them about pulling teeth and about taking care of a woman with tetanus. "I'm going back there this month," I said.

"I make a point of leaving the past in the past," said Nancy Goodman.

"Yes, well, sometimes there are connections with the past that can help you understand the present."

"Well, I just meant, you might be disappointed," she said.

"I know that. I'm not going back to relive memories. I still have friends there. I want to see what's happened to them. It was where I became a doctor, even more than medical school."

"Does that mean we won't have a session when you're gone?" asked the student from Washington.

"Well, I'll either find someone to take my place, or we'll cancel," I said. I walked back to my office, surprised at myself for telling the stories. As I sat at my desk reviewing faculty evaluations by nurses, I began to think about those last days in Mexico, when I was pulling teeth and seeing patients again in the clinic, and how it all ended.

I had begun to gravitate back into the medical consultation room when the dental work slowed. Carl drifted away to a back-room office where he wrote or drew pictures. Our relationship might have been tense had we been forced together, but we barely saw each other. Dr. Silva, the pediatrician from California, returned and was happy to teach me about each patient. His approach was more methodical than Carl's, and he could dissect each piece of a case while Carl seemed to jump to the diagnosis. They both seemed to get to the same place but got there through a different route. More visitors came and went—doctors, dentists, students, and people who wanted to donate money. They would come for a few days, walk around the village, sit in the clinic and watch us work, and then leave. The clinic had become a stop along a mythical counterculture migration trail that seemed to include Big Sur, Taos, Kauai, and Chimaltenango, Guatemala—all places of spiritual growth and alternative models of family, community, and health. It was easy to find the problems in American society and culture, but the solutions were less clear. The village and Carl's project seemed to be a solution. It was remote and exotic and rejected most of the commonly accepted notions of how doctors and patients should behave, which made it all the more interesting to people who mistrusted established systems and hierarchies.

I was becoming tired of all the visitors and my kinship to them as an American volunteer. Even as they rejected materialism and capitalism, they spent their money freely in the village on food, flashlights, and mule rides. The women would hook up with village boys for a few days, while the men attempted to relive old cowboy dreams.

It was almost time for me to return to the United States and begin medical school. I knew I'd miss Ricardo, Rosa, and their family, as well as Luis, Gabriel, and Dr. Silva. As Carl discussed driving back across the border, I decided to travel with him—mostly out of convenience, but also because I wanted one more chance to talk.

It rained all night before my last day at the clinic. The town looked freshly scrubbed. Even the buildings with old faded stucco peeling from adobe blocks seemed to glow. Carl agreed to take me in his Jeep on the way to a meeting about support for a clean-water project. He would drop me off in Texas, where our routes diverged, and I planned to continue by bus. The only problem was that Carl wanted to leave at night because he believed the driving was cooler and easier, and there were fewer police—or maybe he just preferred the night.

As I surveyed the clinic, considering what pictures I should take and how I wanted to remember it, a man, rain still dripping from his plastic poncho, approached me.

"Oiga, oiga," he said.

I listened.

He described a sick relative several hours away in the mountains who could not be moved. Could I accompany him? It wasn't far.

I looked at him—black hair dripping from a straw hat, stubble of beard on his chin, and bloodshot eyes waiting for an answer. He looked familiar, like someone I'd seen before in the clinic. I wanted to tell him it was my last day—that I wasn't really here anymore. In fact, I should already have been traveling back toward my home, away from the mules, the contaminated drinking water, and the pigs that prowled for garbage down alleys. I wanted to tell him to come back later, when I'd be gone.

"I'll ask Dr. Silva and Carl," I said and then looked for them.

"Sure. Go," Carl said. "Silva and I can take care of the clinic. Take a bag with medicines and instruments. You never know what you'll find. We'll leave when you get back."

He was so enthusiastic in helping me prepare for the ride that I had to go, in spite of my own reluctance.

We climbed out of the village and followed the river into the mountains. The trail switchbacked up one ridge, wound down to an arroyo crossing, and then followed the river until a river crossing became necessary. All of the rain from high in the mountains had raised the river level. At the crossing, the mules hesitated as the water came up to the saddles and, in places, up to the mules' necks. My companion laughed as I struggled to hang on and keep dry while my mule stumbled over the river boulders, seeking a secure footing.

After several hours, voracious biting flies landed on the mule, leaving bloody spots where they had bitten into flesh. The mule swished its tail and shook as it tried to defend itself. I found myself thinking that this was just a routine trip up the mountain, yet I was already soaked, and the horse was bleeding. I felt myself losing control as the animal bounded ahead of my guide, up the trail to escape the flies. We reached a cooler, shadier area, where three men with guns suddenly emerged from behind a tree.

With insistent motions, they forced me from the mule and checked my pockets. Meanwhile, my guide arrived and yelled at the men.

"He's a doctor from the clinic. He's just a doctor."

The men stopped and smiled at me. "*Muy bien*, Doctor," they said and helped me to get back on my mule.

"Gracias," I said, shaking, and I felt myself wishing the men had turned us back, so I could go home.

"*De nada*," they said.

We continued in tense silence for a few minutes before my guide explained that there were problems with soldiers in the area, and the men had thought I was with the soldiers. They were his neighbors, and they would not harm us, but we should stay together.

Despite his reassurances I continued to be scared about my safety until we reached the house an hour later. My legs were sore, and my feet were cold and wet. As I admired the log construction of the house, a man emerged to help me dismount, and I recognized him immediately.

"Demetrio," I said. We shook hands and hugged as he explained that his father was sick. It was his older brother who had brought me from the clinic. Demetrio would have come except that the soldiers were still looking for him. He showed me his healing burns and scars with pride and satisfaction, and I nodded. The pattern of the scars on his legs resembled the shapes of continents on the ocean, and he showed them off like new tattoos. It was probably just as well he had not come to the clinic because Carl still remembered the aftermath of Demetrio's escape. But it was nice to see him, here at the end of my long trip. He told me that he felt strong, even strong enough to get his girlfriend Carmen pregnant. He laughed as he told me this and made a gesture with his hands, flexing his arms and fists to demonstrate his vigor. Then he told me they'd be getting married. Did I want to attend the wedding?

"This is my last day," I said. "Tomorrow, I go back to the United States."

"Too bad," he said. "We'll be roasting a pig."

As I approached his father, I smelled pungent folk remedies. It was common for patients to utilize both *curanderos*—traditional healers—and physicians in an attempt to maximize their chances for a cure. I felt the pack of herbs and oils as I pressed on the man's abdomen. A look of surprise and pain registered against a backdrop of stoic denial. Don Luis shook my hand forcefully as he introduced himself. He told me the pain had been increasing over the past three days. He pressed my hand against the area of his abdomen where the pain seemed worst, as if my hand might reach through the skin and squeeze the pain from the diseased organ.

"Your hand cured my grandson," he said, and he pointed to the baby clutching at its mother's breast. There were no signs of the illness or the seizure, and I almost wondered if it was the same baby. It all seemed so long ago.

Perhaps if it hadn't been my last day, I might have gone along—pretended my hand was magical, powerful. But it was my last day, and I just couldn't do it anymore.

"I don't know what's wrong," I said, pulling my hand away.

Demetrio stared at me, disbelieving. They had brought me here for a cure.

"Don't you have a medicine or injection to cure my father?" he asked.

"No."

"But you have your bag of medicine," he said.

"Yes, I brought medicine for pain, diarrhea, ulcers, but I'm not sure what is wrong," I said. "It could be appendicitis. We should take him to the clinic. Dr. Silva and Carlos are there."

"No, he wants to stay home. There are soldiers." Demetrio's eyes pleaded with me insistently. And it scared me.

"Why?" I asked, even as I knew the answer, resisting it, not wanting to participate in the plan.

Demetrio said, "Por favor."

"Your hand, please," said don Luis.

I looked at my hand, and I didn't want to pretend that I was performing some kind of magical cure. I wanted to go home, to get out of the place. But I knew he needed it, wanted it, believed in it, so I put my hand on his stomach where the pain was the worst. He moaned softly as I felt the dry skin that covered whatever was wrong inside. I massaged the stomach slowly, feeling a small lump—perhaps a muscle, perhaps something else. The muscles under the skin yielded to my fingers, slowly relaxing so that I could touch everything inside. After a few minutes, I stopped.

And then I gave Demetrio a bottle of medicine for ulcers and one for diverticulitis and another for kidney stones.

"Try one. If it doesn't work, try the others." I said.

He smiled. "Gracias," he said, satisfied now that I had decided to help, and then he continued to speak. "I have something for Tony. Will you give it to him?"

"Well, he's in the United States, in California, and I'm going to Boston."

"Good, then you can give it to him."

I smiled as I realized that to Demetrio, Boston and California were just the names of places like the small villages along the river: Chilar, where he lived; and Los Árboles, a few miles away.

"Yes, I'll take it to him," I said.

He gave me a handful of seeds.

"What are they?" I asked.

"Seeds of marijuana," he said. "From our plants."

"Well, I don't know," I said.

They were like tiny green pebbles in my hand.

"When Tony took me in his truck, he asked me for seeds so he could grow strong marijuana at his place."

"Bueno," I said, putting the seeds into my pocket. I planned to throw them away when I got out of sight. But for now, I accepted the gift.

After coffee and some beans, I was ready to ride back. Don Luis appeared to be resting. As I was about to mount my mule, I asked Demetrio, "Why do you grow marijuana instead of beans and corn, like everyone else?"

He laughed at me. "Everyone here in Chilar grows marijuana. Come over here for a minute."

I followed him as he walked along a small stream. He pointed out marijuana plants all along the stream.

"It's everywhere in Chilar. We all do it because our land is so steep and the soil so poor. We have to grow it to live. And some people grow opium too. But not us. The soldiers like to take it and sell it themselves, or they take our money, so we fight them," he said. "They take American money; they take our money; and they sell the drugs." Demetrio's tiny log home was not much of an advertisement for the profits of growing marijuana. But maybe it would have been worse without it. I didn't know. So the question of whose story was correct, Demetrio's or Luis's, had been partially solved. I was surprised that Ricardo did not know about his friends and their marijuana.

"Today is my last day," I said to Demetrio. "Tonight I'm going back to the United States. I'll ride down the mountain on a mule and get in a truck and wake up in the United States."

"To the other side," he said. "Go with God. Until the next time." He waved to me as I left.

The ride down the mountain went quickly. The sun was setting, and my mind kept jumping from thought to thought. I almost fell off of my mule for lack of attention to low-hanging branches and dips in the trail. But I hung on to the saddle horn and brushed away the branches. When I arrived at the clinic, Demetrio's brother had already disappeared back up the trail to Chilar. I sat on my mule in the gathering darkness, listening to the flow of men back from the fields to their homes. I lifted my bag of medicines from the saddlebag for the last time and swung my leg over to the ground. Luis emerged from the clinic to greet me, carrying a box to the Jeep.

"Time to go to the other side," he said.

Chapter Seventeen

"*EL OTRO LADO*," THE OTHER SIDE, WAS HOW PEOPLE IN THE village referred to the United States. The term referred to the Rio Grande, which separates much of Mexico from the United States, but *the other side* also meant more. The other side of the world—a mysterious world of dreamlike quality where anything was possible. A world of money, food, and safety, without soldiers, without tragedy and sickness. Anyone who could pass across to the other side was imbued with a special mystique and power. Carl Wilson passed across to the other side several times every year, bringing back medical equipment, books, money, and doctors. He also had the power to take villagers with him, as if he wrapped them in an impenetrable cloak that allowed them to pass only with him. Usually he took children needing operations, but he also took Luis regularly for extra schooling and training, and others might go along to help at fund-raising events or to learn special skills.

As I loaded my clothes into the Jeep, young children gathered around, laughing and smiling, hoping to touch me or one of the others, much as visitors to a space launch watch the astronauts wistfully before they blast into space.

I said my good-byes with a certainty that I would return to this place and these people. Although Ricardo and Rosa shed tears, I maintained an emotional detachment that I didn't understand. Ricardo's arms shook as he hugged me, while Rosa held her fingers to her eyes as if she could change the picture in front of her. Did my tearless eyes prove how I really felt, or was I just drained, focused on escaping all of the demands and needs around me? I occupied my mind with tasks. I put my bag of medicines into the Jeep as if I might need them along the way in the United States.

Carl wanted to drive, and Luis sat next to him, so I jumped into the back with the clothes and boxes. By repositioning boxes, I created a soft nest of blankets and sleeping bags. Once it became clear that Carl was determined to drive all night, Luis and I took turns sleeping in the nest. It made for a bizarrely fragmented night of interrupted dreams, shadows, potholes in the road, and pieces of conversation with Carl.

One went something like this. "I saw Demetrio," I said. "He's growing dope—marijuana. It's all over Chilar."

"Yes, and it's not only Chilar. It's all over the mountains. Fields that used to be corn or beans have become row after row of marijuana. And the villagers are different. Sometimes you'll hear them at night coming through the village, their mules packed down with drugs, hurrying to a rendezvous. Later you can recognize them with their new radios, clothes, and boxes from the city. Soon they'll want cars and electricity. And the federales, those soldiers you see, they take money from everyone—the growers, the buyers, the government."

The Jeep bumped along as we lapsed into thought and memory.

"They all want to either be soldiers or kill soldiers," he said.

"Who?" I asked.

"The boys," he said. "They used to come to the clinic to watch us and learn, but not anymore. Now they have their guns, and they're macho. They think they're grown up. Like that Demetrio."

"Well, but there's Luis," I said. Luis was sleeping in the back.

"Yes, because I've taken an interest in him. Shown him things. His parents have given him to me because they can see what's happening out there."

"They gave him to you?"

"Yes. Told me to take care of him, teach him, like a father. They're old and sick—tuberculosis. Luis has a wild streak, and they knew they couldn't handle him."

"He loves to drive the Jeep," I said, because what I really wanted to say, that real parents don't sleep with their children, would have exploded his fantasy. And as we talked, I felt myself treading close to the line where the truth would come out.

"Oh, there are at least ten families that have asked me to take their sons. And the boys all hang around the Jeep and ask to drive it. But Luis is the only one I've allowed to drive."

The engine hummed, and flashes of roadside dwellings and cracked pavement punctuated our strange conversation. I wondered how many families knew of Carl's other interest in their sons, the sexual interest. I wanted to ask him about it—to see if he would lie or be surprised that I knew, or perhaps engage in a discussion. At least we would be facing the truth. But sometimes the truth was too dangerous to discuss. And Luis was there, and I did not want to embarrass him.

Instead, I said, "I'm not sure I did much good."

"What?"

"I didn't know what I was doing. I acted like I did. And they trusted me, so I started to believe that I knew something. But I didn't really."

"No one does. Read the books. It's all guessing and deception. More patients get better than die, regardless of what the doctor does. And since most people get better, the odds are with you. You just try to improve the odds a little and make the patients a little less frightened of being alone with their illness. Those years of medical school just teach you how to deceive them. Make you believe that you are really responsible for the cure, when it's the people themselves. Medicine is part of the exploitation of the poor. One more way to keep them enslaved, like the banks and the schools and the police do. All part of the oppression of the poor. That's why we need to build our own grain bank, our own water system, our own schools—so that we can put development into the hands of the people. The clinic is only one step."

I thought about it for a while. I hadn't realized I was part of a plan to re-create the village into some kind of socialist cooperative. I had never thought to ask, because the daily medical needs seemed enough, even too much sometimes. But I wondered why Carl was so dedicated and committed to this place. What was it that drove him so relentlessly, so intensely?

"But what do we, I mean as Americans, have to do with it?"

"We're all citizens of the world. Actually, if anything, we are the enemy, and because we know the enemy, we can be more effective. We work on one place and it becomes an example, a model for others. Forget about Americans or Mexicans or Africans. We're all one people, and it's only in our caring about and loving each other that we become a family."

I couldn't answer that. He had formed a comprehensive philosophy that worked for him. I knew he cared about the sick children, the farmers with tuberculosis, and the women with swollen feet, and they trusted him with their lives. He did it all like someone in the family might: without asking for money. But healing people gave him a power over them. A power that drew children toward him, and teenaged boys. And that was what bothered me—not just the boys, but the way it all coalesced. I wanted to understand him and use him as my road map for a good life as a good doctor. I wanted his life to be an example that would contrast with the greed, selfishness, and arrogance that characterized some of the successful doctors I had known. But he had his own selfish interests.

And I wondered if I had my own, if that same power to cure and to know secrets would corrupt me or seduce me. Or perhaps it would be the promise of money, a nice home, a wife—all the pieces of a good life in return for my knowledge and skill as a doctor. No one would criticize me for benefiting from medicine, but would I even remember what I said at my medical school interview? What were my hidden desires? Would I ever try to fulfill them or satisfy them through my position?

Hours later, I was asleep in the back, in the middle of an uneasy dream, when we abruptly stopped. The door swung open, and I heard a police radio. My eyes squinted in the afternoon sunlight as two Texas highway patrolmen told me to stand up. They searched the Jeep and found my bag of medicines.

"What's this?" they asked.

"Medicines," I said. "Tetracycline, ampicillin, Tylenol."

"Are you a doctor?"

"No," I said.

"Are any of you a licensed physician?"

"No." I looked at Carl as he shook his head. I thought that there must be some mistake.

How could he say no? Maybe he had not paid a fee for a license. I waited and waited for an explanation that would satisfy the police and allow us to continue our journey. But there was none. If he was not licensed or not a physician, what was he? And what would happen to me, traveling with him and depending on him?

"You're under arrest for possession of narcotic drugs."

Handcuffs squeezed my wrists behind my back as I backed into the police car for the trip to the jail. As I watched our Jeep disappear from view, I noticed the people stopping on the highway or driving slowly to look at us. I could imagine their thoughts. We were dusty and sweaty. Carl's deeply etched face, scraggly beard, long curly hair and deep-set eyes—bloodshot from driving all night—made him look like a drug addict. His jeans and T-shirt did not suggest he might be a doctor. Luis was the most presentable of the three of us, but his nervousness, his strongly accented English, and his Mexican passport made him suspect. I had been awakened from sleep into a bright daylight search and interrogation without even knowing where I was. I must have looked dazed, frightened, and disheveled. We probably fit the profile of drug smugglers, and the bags of medicine confirmed their suspicions.

At the jail an officer searched my clothes and patted down my legs and head, looking for hidden weapons. Then he pressed my hands and fingers into black ink and fingerprinted me. He removed my belt from my pants, lest I would consider suicide. And then I joined the others in a cell with two bunk-bed springs—no mattresses—and a toilet in the middle of the room.

Finally, away from the police and their scrutiny, I stared at Carl. "Why don't you have a medical license?" I asked. I felt angry and deceived.

"Well, why did you take your bag of medicines with you? That wasn't very smart, was it?" he said.

"I just thought maybe we might need them. They aren't dangerous."

"No, but the police are dangerous. You cannot give them any excuse, no matter how trivial," he said.

"So what about your license?" I asked.

"I don't need it in Mexico, and I don't practice anywhere else," Carl said. "Actually, I'm not a doctor in the usual sense of the word. I've taken classes and had practical experience, but I never graduated from medical school. I came to the village as a tourist and brought along some medicines and bandages. The people convinced me to become their doctor. The medical school allowed me to participate in their physician's assistant program, and then I came back to be their doctor. And that's what I've been. The government ignores me because they can't provide anything for their people. I've brought medicines, X rays, casts, dental equipment. No one asks me about my license."

"But why didn't you tell me before?"

"I'm sure I told you I wasn't an MD. Everyone in the village calls me 'Doctor.' They call you 'Doctor' too, and you never stop them. In fact, we *are* their doctors." I shook my head. He was right. I'd had opportunities to correct patients who called me 'Doctor,' but I allowed it to pass. I had assumed he was a licensed doctor or physician's assistant or something legitimate because of what he did and what everyone said. Maybe someone had told me, and I had not listened. I felt confused and nauseated.

"So we have been treating people all this time without any license. Even though the people are poor and have no other choices, weren't we breaking the law?"

He smiled. "You can see how fair the law is."

I scanned our cell. This was not my vision of where Carl and the clinic would lead me. I felt frightened, but he seemed calm. "Has this ever happened to you before?" I asked.

"No, this is a novel experience for me. But I am confident we will be released. After all, we are completely innocent."

I put my hand into my pocket and felt the marijuana seeds—the gift from Demetrio to Tony. The police had missed them in their search. I whispered to Carl what I had found. His face became grave, almost deathly pale. He whispered for me to flush them down the toilet immediately.

I sat down on the toilet, self-consciously lowering my pants. The toilet had no seat, just a bowl. There was probably some prison safety reason for it, but it felt degrading and dirty. As I pretended to use the toilet, I dropped the seeds into the water and finally flushed. A few seeds disappeared, but others popped back to the surface, bobbing dangerously into view. I pulled my pants up and explained the result to Carl. He nodded and sat down on the toilet, pretending to use it. After a few minutes, he flushed and inspected the result. And then Luis used it. After Luis sat for a while and flushed, he grinned at us.

"No more. It's gone."

The man in the adjoining cell had been watching. He shook his Afro and shrugged his shoulders as he walked over to us.

He stared at us through bloodshot eyes, holding his pants up with his hand in place of the belt that the police must have taken. He hesitated for a moment and then spoke. "You boys have the runs?"

"Yeah, we just came up from Mexico."

"Oh, Mexico. I never go to Mexico. I'm George Brown, the Travelin' Man, but I never go to Mexico. That Mexican tequila, it gives you the runs. You boys been drinking the Mexican tequila?"

"Well, no, not much," I said, trying to be courteous without prolonging the conversation. George Brown's eyes glowed as he listened, and sweat accented the ebony color of his skin. He shook his head and twitched slightly as he talked.

"Yeah, I'm the Travelin' Man. But I don't like them Mexican jails. You just eat beans and them flat tor . . ."

"Tortillas," I said.

"Yeah, that's it. But I ain't going back to Mexico. I get the runs in Mexico from them beans and tortillas and tequila. You need water when you got the runs. Here, take some water." He passed me his metal cup, and I took a sip.

"Thanks," I said. "I'm going to be a doctor. Well, I hope so, if I don't get thrown out of medical school for this." I realized I was shaking, and tears dripped onto my cheek.

"Hey, now, you keep your socks on, you hear me? Now, you just tell that medical school that George Brown said you should get your chance. Ain't nothing wrong with a little tequila. What you boys done, anyway?"

"Nothing. It's all a mistake."

"Yeah, I know what you mean," he said.

I returned to my box spring and lay down. I thought about my parents, how shocked and frightened they'd be. The money they'd have to pay for lawyers instead of medical school tuition. My eyes surveyed the ceiling, gray cement with yellow lines printed like a tic-tac-toe board over it—perhaps a motif to match the bars of the cell. I wondered if this fork in the road would determine my life's path forever. One path led to medical school, residency training, and a life as a physician with money, family responsibilities, and success. The other led to jail and expulsion from medical school, life as a rebel and outcast on the fringes of society, without family. A wanderer, perhaps like George Brown, a travelin' man, but with my pride and dignity. Or perhaps like Carl, I'd find a village and make my own rules. They were extreme paths; perhaps it was fear that drove me to think about them. As I continued to create scenarios for my life paths, a terror filled my mind, and I could barely breathe. Then the morning guard arrived and called our names.

"You can go," said the guard.

"Go? You mean we're free?" I asked.

"Yes, we tested your medicine. No narcotics. We've voided your arrest. You're free. Your vehicle is outside."

They gave us our clothes and let us out. As I was walking away, I looked at George Brown. He was smiling at me, almost laughing. "We going to medical school now. Oooeee!" And he slapped his hand and hopped in the air. "Oh yeah! My boy is goin' to medical school now!"

Chapter Eighteen

I SAT IN MY OFFICE, MY EYES PASSING OVER REPORTS AND memos and finally coming to rest on a stack of faculty evaluations that I needed to review before my meeting with each faculty member. The evaluation meeting was one of the most important parts of my job as chairman because it was the time that we made decisions about faculty goals and salary and figured out what had been accomplished over the past year. I leaned back in my chair and rubbed my neck. It felt sore from not sleeping the right way, and my legs ached.

As I reviewed the faculty evaluations, I was struck by how different our jobs were from my initial expectations. One faculty member was criticized for not billing at a high enough level and not documenting enough on the medical record. Nurses criticized another for spending too much time teaching medical students and residents. On Rick's evaluation, a nurse wrote: "Rick drives me crazy. When we are backed up, he goes out to the waiting room and tells patients there will be an eight-hour wait to be seen. It would be better for everyone if he would just pick up a chart and see the patients and get the workup started." I remembered how patients at our clinic in Mexico would wait all day to see me and never complain. What was the difference? In neither case did patients usually pay for their care. In both cases, we were working as hard as we could. But in Mexico, people did not expect much. They did not believe doctors could change the trajectory of illness, the fate ordained by a higher power. But in our emergency department, everyone expected to be cured, to be treated quickly, and to not suffer.

I did not look forward to my evaluation sessions with the faculty where I would have to read them the critical comments from nurses. As a distraction, I began to write a letter to Ricardo and Rosa informing them of my planned visit. I did not want to show up without an invitation from them. I struggled with my Spanish as I wrote.

Dear Rosa and Ricardo,

I am thinking of coming to the village to visit in the next two to three weeks. Would it be convenient for me to stay with you? I have fond memories of your home and family and, of course, the clinic. My wife will be not be accompanying me.

Best wishes to all,
David

I did not want to say too much about what was happening in my life and why I wanted to visit. We could talk about it when I arrived. I imagined Rosa and Ricardo and their children greeting me with delight and surprise, like the arrival of an unexpected package.

Then I checked my e-mail. There were the usual messages from the dean and from various faculty members about upcoming retreats, budget problems, trading shifts, meeting announcements, and articles and memos to review. I came upon a strange one from a woman named Peggy Norman.

Dr. Sklar,

I wanted to tell you how impressed I was with your comments at the medical executive committee meeting. You were the only person there who was willing to face the truth about our dismal financial situation and tell us that we need to change what we are doing or the hospital and medical school will go bankrupt. It's not a pretty picture, but it is the truth. I have been feeling this need to change in my clinic for quite some time, but anytime I said it, people said I was crazy and told me to just calm down and not get so worked up. But you said what I have been thinking, and now I'm still nervous about it, but at least I don't think I'm crazy.

Sincerely,
Peggy Norman, MD

I reread her comments and smiled. At least my comments at the executive committee a week ago had reached one receptive set of ears. I knew that the dean and administrators had been annoyed. They did not like to have bad news discussed in public meetings. Those meetings were for morale boosting and positive reports. But I was tired of our refusal to face the reality of our situation, so when the chief of nursing reported that the nursing shortage had been solved by closing beds, I had to talk about how overcrowded the emergency department was and how anyone with insurance would never wait the five hours it would take to be seen. Only uninsured, indigent patients with no choice would do that, and we could not have a hospital if only indigent patients could get into it.

I looked again at the name, Peggy Norman, and tried to remember who she was and what she looked like.

I felt too distracted to read more evaluations, work on my articles, read more e-mails, or do any other productive work, so I decided to go home.

When I got home, there was a man waiting for me at the gate. He had on a tie and sports jacket, and his face looked faintly familiar.

"Hi," he said. "My name is Felix. Beautiful place you have here."

"Come in," I said. "What can I do for you?"

"Well, I have to say, I've always admired this property. The house surrounded by cottonwood trees in the middle of what is it, about three acres?"

"Yes," I said. "It's beautiful. It is so peaceful."

"Well, let me get to the point. One of my friends told me you are going through some personal difficulties. Now, I've been through a divorce myself, and I know what it can be like. It knocks you for a loop. And financially it is a nightmare. Dividing everything up, child custody, and lawyers. It's a mess. So I wanted you to know that I'm interested in buying your house. No pressure. But in case it is something you decide to do, I could spare you the need to hire a real estate agent. Then we can both win. You get an easy sale and pay no commission, and I get a better deal on the house because you don't need to sell it for such a high price. How does that sound?"

I realized I had seen this man on television. He was a news anchor, and he had a wonderful, deep, resonant voice that made you immediately trust him and believe that the news he was telling was true and important. He had dyed black hair brushed back and a pink, fleshy face with perfect white teeth that seemed to be perpetually smiling. "I . . . I don't know. I didn't realize people knew about my situation. I haven't told many people yet. And even my kids. They are at camp now, and we've barely started to talk about it."

"Well, you'd be amazed what the neighbors notice. A moving truck that carts off a bunch of furniture. A car no longer in the driveway. People notice these things. Over the years, when I covered murders, I'd often find that the neighbors were quite observant of even the smallest details. They'd tell me things that even the police did not know. So could I take a look around?"

I took him into the kitchen, and he put his hands on the counters. "We'd need to recover these," he said. "Granite would look nice."

We moved into the living room.

It was thick adobe with wood vigas in the ceiling. "This room stays cool even in the summer," I said. "The cottonwood trees provide wonderful shade."

We moved into the bedrooms. "Excuse the mess. I just worked a night shift in the ER and had to sleep all day so the bed's a mess."

"ER doc?" he said. "Now that's a job that must be interesting. Maybe you'd like to come on the news sometime and tell people about it. You know that's what I do. I'm the newscaster for Channel 4."

"Yes, I thought I recognized you."

He moved through the other bedrooms, out into the portal and the yard, occasionally stopping to feel the adobe or rub his hand along a wall.

"Yes," he said. "This is just what I'm looking for. How much do you want for it?"

"Well, I'm not sure. I mean, I don't even know if I want to sell it."

"Well, just give me a ballpark?"

"Oh, I don't know, maybe six hundred thousand."

"Oh, well, that's a good starting point. I might be able to go $575,000. Do we have a deal?"

My head was spinning. I wanted to throw him out and go to sleep and make all of the events of the past weeks disappear. But it was so much money, and it would allow Laura and me to buy our own houses, and I wouldn't have to pay that huge mortgage. "I . . . I'll have to think about it," I said, weak and almost out of breath.

I showed him to the gate.

"Here's my number. Call me after you think about it. Great meeting you," he said.

I staggered back to my bedroom and threw myself on the bed. I could feel tears welling up in my eyes. I'd have to talk to Laura about this. What if she wanted to do it? Where would we live? Suddenly, I imagined myself homeless, out on the streets like many of my patients. I could probably manage, but what about the kids? My life was not supposed to turn out this way. When I had returned from Mexico and started medical school, I thought I had set a secure course that would continue as long as I worked at it. This was not part of the plan. As I buried my head in the pillow, I thought about medical school and residency and the decisions I had made and how they seemed to flow naturally from what I did in Mexico, from the values and lessons I had learned there. Or perhaps I had been co-opted by health-care business imperatives like most of the doctors that Carl met. As I lay there, I suddenly had an image of myself and my life as a meal being consumed by ants—ants that crawled over it and through it, picking it apart, and digesting the pieces. And I found myself retreating again, retracing the journey of how I had gotten here.

Chapter Nineteen

WHEN I RETURNED FROM MEXICO, I ENTERED MEDICAL school with both an advantage and a disadvantage over my class-mates. My advantage was my familiarity with the diseases with long complicated names. I had seen cases of hepatitis and had treated a woman with tetanus, a baby with tuberculosis, and a musician with diabetic ketoacidosis. I had listened to lungs, heard crackles, seen pus on tonsils, and felt a seizure. My disadvantage was that I realized I could make a diagnosis and treat a problem without knowing the name of the muscle or nerve involved, without memorizing biochemi-cal reactions or drug kinetics, without wearing a white coat or holding a stethoscope. But my professors expected me to memorize the nerves of the brachial plexus and the enzymes of the biochemical metabo-lism of sugar and to display my knowledge at the bedside of a patient whom I had never met, while surrounded by twenty other white-coated medical students. We called it making rounds, and we would follow an esteemed professor from interesting case to interesting case like a swarm of pigeons following a trail of crumbs, stopping to place our twenty stethoscopes over a chest to hear a murmur or to place our fingers over a thyroid gland. I struggled to fit in, to learn the rituals and the facts even as I doubted their importance. I thought I had a better way, one that fit newer educational theories and followed naturally from my Mexico experience. I wanted to immerse myself in clinical work with real patients right from the beginning and relate their prob-lems to the microbiology or biochemistry I needed to know. A patient with tuberculosis would lead me to the study of mycobacteria and the antibiotics needed to cure the infection. Pharmacology could become relevant as diseases or injuries in real patients required knowledge of the drugs that could provide relief or cure.

I gravitated to a farmworkers' clinic where my Spanish fluency and my familiarity with the culture and belief systems of the patients made me particularly valuable. I found the role of assisting a volunteer doctor familiar and rewarding. Although I could only go to the clinic occasionally, it helped me maintain my vision of the kind of medicine I wanted to practice and the kind of doctor I wanted to be. One day, I remember, a man came to the clinic with diarrhea and vomiting.

"What have you been doing today?" I asked as part of the history.

"Working. Working in the fields."

"What do you do in the fields?" I asked.

"I spray."

"What? What do you spray?"

"I spray for insects."

"Do you wear any protective clothing—goggles, a mask, a special suit of clothes?"

He shook his head. "No, they told me I only need protective clothes if I spray for more than one hour. So I stopped after one hour."

We sent him to the emergency department to be treated for pesticide poisoning. When he left in an ambulance, I remember his face alternately looking back at us and looking forward at the street leading to the hospital. I wondered who would pay the bill, and what the treatment might be. A few weeks later, I returned to the farmworkers' clinic and found a cabbage with a note informing me that he had received an antidote injection, and everything was fine, and he would not spray again.

I wanted to practice where it didn't matter whether a patient was rich or poor, insured or uninsured, educated or uneducated, living on an estate or homeless. I wanted to be able to wear jeans, scrubs, or a shirt and tie with a white coat and not have it matter to anyone how I looked or sounded. The only thing that would matter would be the skill and knowledge and commitment to care and help that I would bring to the patient encounter, and we would just be two people, two equals, except that one was helping the other. At the farmworker clinic, everyone—even the doctors—helped mop the floor, clean the counters, and put away the donated medicines. And patients brought artichokes and huge green heads of lettuce for the nurses and doctors. At first I thought that I would become a general practitioner with broad skills that I could take with me wherever I might want to work in the world—a clinic, a hospital, or office. But general practitioners were becoming family medicine doctors and concentrating on outpatient practices, offices, and patients with diabetes or high blood pressure who needed prescription refills and adjustments. Although the variety appealed to me, the challenge of making a diagnosis and doing something important seemed to be missing.

After completing my courses in anatomy, physiology, pathology, biochemistry, and pharmacology, I began my formal clinical training in the hospital. Even with my experience in Mexico, I was not prepared for the demands of rapid assessment and integration of basic science with actual patients. I began my first rotation in the hospital in a course known as Physical Diagnosis. Pairs of medical students were assigned to a senior physician who would provide mentorship in the skills of physical diagnosis. I was paired with Jenny Beal, a talkative, enthusiastic woman. Jenny had long straight blond hair, which hung almost to her waist. We drove together to the hospital to meet our preceptor, Dr. Abbott, an eminent gastroenterologist who had an excellent reputation as a teacher.

Jenny said, "I'm so nervous. I've never examined anyone before, except when we practiced on ourselves two weeks ago."

"Don't worry. You'll do fine," I said.

"Aren't you nervous?" she asked.

"No, not really. I examined a lot of people when I worked in Mexico. I'm just hoping I haven't forgotten everything I learned." But I *was* nervous, because what I had been doing in Mexico was not complete. It was a fragment of a physical exam, enough to make a possible diagnosis but not enough for medical school.

We put on our white coats as we entered the hospital. My white coat hung clumsily from my shoulders, reaching to my knees. I stuffed my stethoscope into the huge side pocket along with a red, rubber reflex hammer and a vibrating fork. Jennifer's white coat tucked and flared in just the right places and looked more like a designer dress than a laboratory jacket.

Dr. Abbott was waiting for us in the internal medicine conference room. He stood to greet us, and I noticed that his moustache wiggled nervously. He had combed his scarce blond hair from the sides over his hairless middle scalp. He described our assignment—his personal patients carefully chosen because of interesting physical findings and history. "And don't forget the medical history," he said. "It may be the clue to the diagnosis. You will be graded upon the completeness of your history and physical examination. And you must do a complete physical exam."

"Complete?" I asked. "Does that mean . . ." I stopped, searching for the appropriate term.

"Complete, Mr. Sklar, means complete. It includes the rectal exam and the genital exam."

I nodded and noticed that Jenny was frowning at me. We had heard that Dr. Abbott emphasized the rectal exam because, as a gastroenterologist, he often treated patients with colon cancer who might have been diagnosed earlier if a doctor had performed a rectal exam. "I've found more cancer by doing a rectal exam than by performing any other part of the physical exam," he said. His tired eyes bulged out of puffy sockets as he emphasized his words and held up his hand to demonstrate the length of his index finger.

He read off our assignments. My patient was named Howard Zigler, in room 302. Jenny got Napoleon White.

"You'll have one-half hour, and then we will reconvene here for your presentations."

I hurried off to the third floor and pushed open the heavy yellow door of room 302. The room reeked of urine and antiseptic soap. Two beds jutted out from the window in parallel, and I stood at the foot of the first bed staring at an obese man breathing into an oxygen mask. Fortunately, Mr. Zigler was in the other bed. He was a small, muscular man with a high forehead and dark sideburns, and his skin had a pale, sallow sheen.

"Hello, Mr. Zigler," I said cheerfully. "I'm David Sklar, a medical student. Your doctor asked me to give you a physical and ask you a few questions."

"I already got my physical," he said.

"Yes, I know that. I need to give you another physical."

"Another physical? What for? They already checked me inside and out. They know my heart is shot and my kidneys are gone. What are you gonna do for me?"

"Well, I'm just learning to become a doctor. I need to—"

"Practice?" he interrupted. "You want to practice on me?"

"Well, it's not exactly practice. I've actually taken care of real sick people myself in Mexico," I said.

"You a Mexican?"

"No."

"So what are you?" he asked.

"I'm Jewish," I said.

"Oh, Jews are smart. That's why they all have money. Never spend it either. Cheap bastards. Nothing personal against you, but you know what I mean."

I sighed. I resented Mr. Zigler for making this hurdle in my medical school career so difficult. "OK, Mr. Zigler, so do you mind if I ask you some questions and do a physical?"

"OK, as long as you don't do that finger-up-the-butt thing again," he said.

I hesitated, considering my response. Without the rectal exam, my physical would not be complete. "Mr. Zigler," I said, "I realize that the rectal exam is unpleasant, but it's one of the ways we can detect cancer."

"You go near me with that finger, and that's the last time you'll see that finger," he said, making his eyes large and voice loud to emphasize his resolve.

"Well, then, let's move on to some basic questions. Now, Mr. Zigler, what brought you to the hospital?"

"Brought me? To the hospital? My ex-wife, Tammy, brought me."

"No, I mean what is your chief complaint," I said, taking out a pad of paper to record his answer.

"Complaint? Television—you can only get one channel," and he pressed a button near his bed to demonstrate the poor reception of his television. "That's my complaint. And the food."

I looked at my watch. Already ten minutes had been wasted. I was supposed to complete my history and physical and then organize it for presentation to Dr. Abbott.

I tried a shortcut. "Mr. Zigler, do you know what's wrong with you? I mean, what did the doctors say?"

"Well, if I tell you, wouldn't that be cheating?"

"No, Mr. Zigler. You can tell me."

He stared into my eyes to see if I would flinch, perhaps look down at the floor and admit that I was cheating, trying to win the game without following the rules. But I locked my gaze upon his, noticing how red and bloodshot his eyes were. His nose lay flattened and bent to the left, and a thick scar twisted above and through his left eyebrow.

"OK," he said. "The hell of it all is that I'm dying. They won't come out and say it, but my kidneys are shot, and my heart is failing. They want me to go on dialysis, but I don't want it, so now they want me to see a goddamned headshrinker to see if I'm nuts."

"Why don't you want the dialysis?"

"It's personal. Let's just leave it at that."

"Well, how did you get to this point?" I asked.

"Too much booze and women," he said.

I looked over my list of questions. Under the heading of "Past Medical History" were questions about alcohol use and marital history.

"How much do you drink?" I asked.

"About a case," he said.

"A case a week?" I asked.

"No, a case of Bud every day. Usually I have about a six-pack for breakfast. I mix beer with orange juice. You ever try that?"

"No," I said.

"You ought to. That way, you get your vitamins."

I wondered how anyone could drink so much beer. I felt bloated after two cans.

"And how about your social situation?" I asked. "Are you married?"

"I'm between wives," he said.

"So you're divorced," I said.

"Yeah, been divorced three times. But hell, I ain't learned. I'm gonna marry my nurse here if I can get out long enough. Do you know her—Annie McCormick?" He looked up at me hopefully as I continued to write.

"No. No, I don't know her. I'm just a medical student. But congratulations."

"You married?" he asked.

"No. No, I'm not," I said.

"Didn't think so," he said.

"Why?" I asked. "Why didn't you think so?"

"You seem kind of tense, like you're not gettin' any. You better not wait too long."

"Well, Mr. Zigler, with all the studying I have to do in medical school it's difficult to find the time . . ." I drifted off.

"Now that's bullshit, if ever I heard it," he said, and his face turned a reddish gray. He sat up as if he were ready to punch me. "I'm gonna tell you about my second wife, Maura. I met her when I was married to my first wife, Suzette. I'd get together with her at lunch, and we'd get a motel room. I'd see her on Saturday when Suzette went shopping. We had to be together even though there wasn't any time. We had to touch each other and smell each other's skin. It was like eating and breathing, just no choice in it. So don't you go telling me about not having no time."

"Well, maybe you're right; I guess I haven't found the right one yet."

"You gotta be looking. They don't just fall from the sky into your lap. And when you see one, then you gotta treat her right—buy her flowers, perfume, and dresses. You got a lot to learn Mr. Smart-ass Jew medical student," he glared at me.

Much as I wanted to ignore his ramblings as the disordered thoughts of a chronic alcoholic, I also knew there was some truth to what he said. The demands of medical school were a convenient excuse for withdrawing from the emotional whirlwind created by the words *I love you*. And I had yet to say them. I had never bought flowers or perfume for anyone. Sometimes I wondered if I'd ever be able to find love and make a commitment. His words seemed to singe my hair and skin, and I felt myself curling up as I continued. "So why did you divorce her?" I asked.

"Which one?" he asked.

"Maura. If you needed to be together all the time, why did you get divorced?"

He shrugged and sighed. "Oh, Maura. Once we got married, it changed. We started fighting. See this." He showed me the scar above his eyebrow. "She did it—threw a plate at me." He became thoughtful and quiet. "She tried to kill me."

"Well, Mr. Zigler, I need to examine you. My time is running out. Do you mind if I listen to your heart and lungs?"

"No, go right ahead." He pulled up his T-shirt for me. His abdomen protruded from his deep chest like a watermelon. I hadn't noticed it under his hospital robe. He became embarrassed as I stared. "I'm gonna lose it before I marry Annie. I promised her." He smiled.

His heartbeat was like the drum of a jazz percussionist with interposed jolts and sudden runs of high-speed softer tones. His lungs gurgled as he took a breath. I might have been concerned if I had been in Mexico, but I knew this was a game, that my findings were unimportant. No one would care.

I wrote down the findings as I heard the overhead announcement requesting that I return to the medicine conference room.

"Mr. Zigler, I have to go now. I've enjoyed getting to know you," I said.

"So what do you think?" he asked.

"About what?"

"How much time have I got?"

"Well, I don't know, but if they are recommending dialysis, you probably need it. People can live a long time on dialysis, but without it . . ."

"Dead," he said. "What's it like dying from your kidneys?"

"I'm not sure. I think your blood gets filled up with all the toxic stuff that should be in your urine, and eventually you go into a coma and your heart stops."

He seemed to consider what I told him, before he said, "So I'll die of piss poison. But it will be my own piss." He smiled at me. "Hey, let's have a beer sometime, if I ever get out of here." I nodded to him as I collected my papers and hurried to the conference room.

Jenny and Dr. Abbott were waiting for me. I listened enviously to Jenny's presentation of her patient, Napoleon White.

"Mr. White is a seventy-one-year-old black male from Mississippi, who presented with chest pain, nausea, vomiting, and sweatiness for one hour. The pain felt like a heavy weight on his chest. He smoked two packs per day and has diabetes. His physical exam revealed congestive heart failure and pulmonary fluid. His electrocardiogram demonstrated the findings of an acute anterior infarction."

"Well, that was excellent," said Dr. Abbott. "I really didn't expect you to include the EKG interpretation, since we have not covered it yet. That was complete and focused. Excellent, excellent." He took her notepapers, and his head bobbed like a chicken as he repeated himself. "Excellent, excellent." Then he looked at me. "And now you, Mr. Sklar."

"Mr. Zigler is a fifty-five-year-old Caucasian male, who presented with renal failure and heart failure due to alcoholism," I said.

Dr. Abbott interrupted me. "Does alcoholism cause kidney failure?"

"I don't know. I haven't had a chance to look it up," I said.

"Well, it doesn't."

"Oh," I said. "He's hoping to marry his nurse, and he drinks a case of beer every day, but he tries to make it nutritionally balanced by mixing it with orange juice."

"That's the most ridiculous thing I've ever heard," said Dr. Abbott. "All right, what did you find on physical exam?"

"He had an irregular heart rhythm that sounded like African drums answering each other in the jungle."

"Very creative description, Mr. Sklar. And what did the rectal exam show?"

"I didn't do the rectal," I said.

"Your grade will reflect that," he said and dismissed us.

Jenny and I drove back to the medical school from the hospital. "Don't worry about the rectal," she said.

"Easy for you to say."

"Well, let me tell you what happened to me. I was examining Mr. White. I was doing the complete exam and touched his penis and scrotum, and he got excited, got an erection. I was so embarrassed. I apologized to him, and he said, 'Now, little lady, nothing to apologize for. This is the first time I've had that happen in ten years. Didn't think it was working anymore, so I'm much obliged.'"

"Magic fingers," I said, and we laughed.

I ran into Dr. Abbott at a conference at the end of the physical-diagnosis course, and that was how I found out what happened to Mr. Zigler. Mr. Zigler had continued to refuse dialysis. He signed out of the hospital against medical advice and married a nurse. She brought him back three days later in a coma, and he died. The hospital was considering whether to discipline the nurse.

I nodded as Dr. Abbott told me the story.

"I don't understand why Mr. Zigler refused dialysis," he said.

"He didn't want to live like that," I said, "hooked to a machine, tubes connected to his arms—that wouldn't be a life for him."

Dr. Abbott seemed uncomfortable with my comment. He flexed his fingers into a fist and looked past me at the dean's photo on the wall. I was sure he could not understand anyone choosing death over life on dialysis. In his world, Mr. Zigler and his diagnosis were identical, and the treatment was clear. But I had watched people in Mexico choose death at home over an uncertain outcome at a hospital. And I had watched them die surrounded by family, in their own bed in their own house in their own village. I felt certain that Mr. Zigler had died happy, with the memory of his nurse blotting out everything else. Dr. Abbott finally opened his hand—his speculations and thoughts about Mr. Zigler over—and said, "Very well," as he turned and walked briskly down the hall.

Chapter Twenty

AS A STUDENT AT STANFORD MEDICAL SCHOOL, I HAD THE opportunity to observe faculty physicians, residents, and other medical students. I would sometimes hear the medical team tell jokes about a patient during hallway discussions, only to watch the team enter the patient's room with a false, exaggerated respectfulness. Hallway uncertainties about treatment would be transformed into certainties during conversations with the patient. I remembered the many conversations with Carl about medical school, and how he had advised against attending, because of these same attitudes and behaviors. Perhaps his decision to practice medicine without the corrupting influence of a medical degree was not so strange.

I tried to minimize the socialization effects of medical school education upon my perspective by choosing medical rotations in county hospitals that focused on poor, uninsured populations. But even in those hospitals, I rarely encountered physicians who questioned the traditional roles of nurses and doctors, the impact of fee-for-service medicine, or the power relationships between patients and the healthcare system. Doctors had their own bathrooms, their own dining room, and their own parking spaces. Patients had to sit and wait while the doctor talked to his wife on the phone about dinner plans. When another doctor came by, they would converse together as if the patients had become invisible. In Mexico, at least we rode the same horses, ate the same food, slept in the same uncomfortable cots, drank the same water, smelled equally bad, and bathed in the same swimming hole. When someone was sick, we were more like a neighbor who happened to have pills and books on hand than a member of royalty with special privileges and protections. Only doctors who had suffered an illness seemed to understand the gap between the world of the doctor and that of the patient, and even for them the differences were moderated because of professional courtesy. I moved from pediatrics to psychiatry to internal medicine to surgery attempting to learn the unique skills and perspectives of each discipline. What I found most difficult was not the patients and their problems, but the faculty physicians and the residents who would show off their knowledge, making fun of the medical students or ignoring them and barely acknowledging the humanity and individual needs of the patients. Even if we didn't know as much in Mexico, we took time with the patients and tried to understand them, as well as their illnesses.

When it came time to choose an internship and residency, I chose to specialize in internal medicine. It was a broad specialty that focused on difficult diagnoses in adult patients. I enjoyed the challenge of putting together clues from lab tests and physical exams. And I thought internal medicine would give me a broad perspective that would be useful wherever I practiced. I selected the University of New Mexico Hospital in Albuquerque for my internship and drove all night to get there. I passed over the mountains and found the land opening up into a great expanse of desert and sky. The green and blue of the California coast transformed into the gray and brown of the Southwest desert. Four years of medical school, and finally, when someone called me "Doctor," it would be true. I was nervous and excited as I started my internship. I was ready to be a doctor, to work one hundred hours a week, to put my patients before everything else, and to finally get paid.

I wore yellow running shoes for the first day of my internship. They were the kind of yellow that calls attention to itself, like the yellow line down the middle of a street. They made me feel light on my feet, the way you want to feel at the start of a race. The internship was the beginning of a long-distance race, all of us standing around nervously early in the morning, wondering if we'd be standing at the end, wondering where the trouble would be—a stomachache, exhaustion, or a wrong turn. The other interns wore ties, pressed shirts, black leather shoes. They were all men and all married, dressed by their wives, and one even carried a lunch sack packed by his spouse. I wore a plain cotton jersey, khaki pants, and my yellow shoes. I was experiencing abdominal cramps and diarrhea from amebiasis, which I had contracted from unclean drinking water during a recent visit to Guatemala, and had to make frequent and sudden trips to the bathroom.

The chairman of internal medicine introduced himself and welcomed us to our internship in Albuquerque, New Mexico. "Two *q*'s and three *u*'s," he said after spelling Albuquerque.

"I realize the brown of the desert may shock many of you who come from greener places," he said. "But the brown grows on you. Anyway, with all the clinical responsibilities you will have as interns, you won't be outside very much." He smiled at us knowingly.

"You should wear your white coats at all times," he said. "Patients expect it. You're doctors now. And a tie. That's my only dress-code requirement. A tie shows a professional attitude." He stared at me. I felt naked and embarrassed. I had chosen the jersey because of the hundred-degree heat. I knew I would be on night call and working for thirty-six straight hours, and I didn't want to overheat. Then he saw my shoes, flashing at him like a caution sign. "Those shoes are very . . . bright," he said, frowning.

"Yes, sir," I said.

Then he gave us our assignments. We were teamed up with medical students, faculty attending physicians, and residents who had completed the internship and were to assist us and oversee our work. Rick was my resident. He was younger and wilder then. He wore wire-rimmed glasses and already had a thick beard that reminded me of Jerry Garcia. He lifted his eyebrows as he cautioned me. "Those yellow shoes—the chief doesn't like your yellow shoes," he said, laughing.

"Should I go home and change?" I asked.

"No. No, of course not. We already have patients. They'll never notice. Here's your list." And he gave me a list of my patients. Some of them had been in the hospital for days or weeks and had a tentative diagnosis written after their names. Others were new patients, just admitted. *Judy Shore* and *Annie Fragua* were two such names that lay on my card like eggs frying on a griddle waiting for a hungry customer.

"Go see each one and write a note about how they're doing," he said. "I'll be in the unit."

I wondered what the unit was but was afraid to ask and expose my ignorance. So I nodded silently and set off to find my patients.

I stopped at a bathroom, hoping to head off a rush of diarrhea that might disrupt my first patient interview, when a huge woman in white and a curved cap stopped me. "That's the patient bathroom," she said. "The doctors' bathroom is over there." She pointed toward the end of the hall. "You are a doctor, aren't you?" she said.

"Yes, I'm David Sklar," I said.

"Well, Doctor Sklar, I'm Pat, the head nurse." She squeezed my hand. "You interns get younger every year."

I smiled and hurried off to the doctors' bathroom. The two stalls were both occupied, and I was about to turn and walk out when a beeper went off. "Oh, shit," someone said, and then the stall door poked open. "Hey, you!" shouted a man in blue scrubs. "Go to room 504; there's a code blue, and I'm stuck here." He handed me his beeper in case further information might follow. "Run!" he yelled.

I ran to room 504 and found a nurse doing cardiopulmonary resuscitation on an obese, elderly woman. The nurse looked at me expectantly.

"She was eating breakfast and coded," the nurse said.

"OK," I said, trying to think.

She pointed at the defibrillator.

"Do you want to shock her?" she said.

I had never used a defibrillator before, though I had seen them used. I knew they were dangerous because of the large jolts of electricity that came out of the paddles. "OK," I said and grabbed the paddles.

"All clear," said the nurse, releasing the patient and waiting for me to do something. I pushed a red button, but nothing happened.

"You have to charge them," she said as she resumed pumping on the patient's chest and blowing into her mouth.

I pressed the charge button and then tried again as the nurse yelled, "Clear!" This time the patient's arms jumped into the air, and I smelled the odor of burnt flesh from the paddles.

"I feel a pulse," said the nurse as the doctor who had been on the toilet arrived.

"Good job," he said as he took the defibrillator paddles out of my hands. "Go call the unit." I went to the nurse's desk in a daze and told them the woman in room 504 needed the unit. The clerk at the desk dialed a number and then gave me the phone.

"Hi," I said. "I'm Doctor Sklar. The woman in room 504 just had a cardiac arrest. She now has a pulse."

The nurse at the other end of the phone told me to hold and passed the phone to Rick, my resident.

"This is Rick," he said.

"Oh, hi. I just resuscitated a woman from room 504. They told me to call the unit."

"Well, that must be some kind of record, a save in your first hour as an intern. Is she one of ours?"

"No, a guy in the bathroom had his pager go off and sent me there."

"Well, good work. Tell the nurse to send her to the unit, and go see your own patients. I'm glad she's not one of ours. We don't need any more unit players."

"OK, thanks," I said and rechecked my card to see if the woman in room 504 was on it. Fortunately, she was not. I took one more look into the room and noticed that by now other doctors and nurses had arrived and were all clustered around the patient. The resident from the bathroom was giving orders to the nurse, and I returned his beeper as he stared up at the monitor. Then I headed off to meet my first patient without a diagnosis next to her name, Judith Shore.

Judith Shore stared at me as I entered her room and seemed to ponder me for a moment before screaming, "Yellow shoes, yellow shoes!" I noticed that the white parts of her eyes were jaundiced, like the color of my shoes, and her skin had a bronze tint. Judith Shore had short black hair, which curled at her neck, and her arms were tied to the bed rails with white Kerlix bandages.

"Yellow shoes, yellow shoes," she said.

I started wondering about my decision to come to Albuquerque and whether I really wanted to do this internship. New Mexico had seemed like the right place—a hospital dedicated to the care of the poor, a place where I could use my Spanish language skills, a land of stark mountains and turquoise sky. But I had not anticipated this. Maybe I could just go back to Carl's clinic, help out in the village. Carl had warned me that doctors were not the solution to the health-care needs of the poor in the developing world because they would pursue their own enrichment and forget about the poor. If I completed the internship, I'd be one of them, a licensed doctor.

"Miss Shore," I said. "I'm your doctor."

"Yellow shoes," she repeated.

Pat, the head nurse, came up behind me. "She doesn't like your shoes," she said. "And neither do I."

I nodded. "I think she's delirious."

We stared at each other for a moment, and then I began to examine Judith Shore. She was more like an animal than a person as she pulled away from me, resisting my probing fingers, pulling against her bandages. Sweat formed upon her forehead in droplets, and her eyes became wild. About halfway through the examination, Rick appeared. "Let's write some orders," he said.

We sat at the doctors' and nurses' station, a group of four chairs behind a long, white counter with a telephone and piles of medical records in the corner.

"She looks terrible," I said.

"It's liver failure, from drinking. She's going to die," he said.

I wrote *hepatitis* next to diagnosis and wondered how my resident knew she was going to die. But I didn't ask.

Our orders were for fluids and sedation but no treatments for her liver. "Isn't there anything we can do for her hepatitis?" I asked.

"No," said Rick. "I think I saw something about steroids in a journal article, but they didn't work. It's her own fault. We're wasting our tax dollars on her, because she'll go out and drink again if we save her. She's a county indigent, so you and I are paying her bill. Anyway, you've got another patient to work up and eight more to see and write notes on."

"Don't some of them stop?" I asked.

"Oh shit, a bleeding-heart liberal," said Rick as he walked away.

I finished my orders and made a mental note to look up hepatitis in the library and find the article about steroids.

I moved to my next patient, Annie Fragua, a thirty-year-old Navajo woman with leukemia. She had received chemotherapy, and now her bone marrow had stopped producing white cells, red cells, and platelets. Any cut would continue to bleed because without platelets, the blood would not clot. Any infection would spread throughout the body because there were no white cells to contain it. We could give platelets and red cells intravenously, but there were no supplies of white cells, so I had to be particularly careful to identify any sign of an infection.

Annie and I talked about her illness.

"I feel weak," she said. "I can't take care of my little girl." She showed me a picture of her three-year-old daughter.

"We'll give you more red cells," I said. "We just have to get you through until your bone marrow starts working again."

She smiled at me and closed her eyes, retreating into her own space.

"I'm going to examine you now," I said.

"OK," she whispered.

I looked everywhere for infection—her feet, her throat, her ears, her teeth, and finally, after an hour, I declared her to be safe. "No infection," I said.

"Thank you."

"Now I have to start an intravenous line in your arm to give you blood and platelets," I said.

She extended her arm and I noticed the purple bruises where previous attempts to put needles into her veins had failed. I held a needle with a catheter in my right hand and searched her arm for a vein that might accept it, a vein that was big enough and straight enough to allow a catheter to slide along its fragile walls without breaking. I found a vein on the back of her hand that looked promising and punctured her dark, soft skin before sliding the needle forward into the vein. Blood began to drip from the catheter, and I connected a plastic tube and taped the catheter in place.

"Thank you," she said.

"I . . . you're welcome," I said and rushed off to tell the nurse that Annie Fragua was now ready for the blood transfusion.

Every day for a month, this sequence of events was repeated. The exam, the search for a vein, the attempts to put a catheter into the vein, and the transfusion.

It became more and more difficult to find a vein. Sometimes I'd look for hours. Finally, I'd go by the feel of my fingertips, like a diviner seeking water in a desert. We'd sit together in quiet desperation, just wanting one more vein, one more transfusion, one more day, checking her blood counts to see if the bone marrow had recovered. She knew before I did that it was not going to happen. She sent for the medicine man and had a ceremony in her room.

"Now, it will come back," I said after her ceremony, as we sat together. She didn't want to give up because of her little girl.

"She needs me," she said.

Finally, a blue spot on her tongue killed her. The infection spread into her blood, and without white cells she was defenseless. The antibiotics that I flushed through her veins could not stop it. I knew that the struggle was hopeless, that the bone marrow would never come back, that this end was inevitable, but she was my first patient to die since I had become a doctor. In Mexico it had been different, because I wasn't really a doctor yet, and I was not in a real hospital with nurses and specialists to help me. But when Annie died, I felt betrayed, as if someone had been playing a joke on me and Annie. I sat with her as the room filled with specialists and nurses summoned for the final moments. As I watched their frantic activity, I found myself wanting to protect her body from them.

Judith Shore was still alive a month later. I had looked up the article on steroids for hepatitis and convinced Rick that we should try it. Her response was slow, almost imperceptible at first, but gradually it became evident that she was getting better. Her color changed until she became a pale ghostly figure speaking in words, then sentences, and finally she had a conversation with me.

"I want to go home," she said. "I'm going to stop drinking."

"You're still sick," I said. "You almost died." It was true, but she was better now.

"I did? I don't remember," she said. "I don't remember anything. Except those shoes. Those yellow shoes."

"I don't wear them anymore," I said.

I sent Judith home a few days later. I saved her card with the diagnosis of hepatitis along with my other cards from that first week. They were souvenirs, like the baseball cards I had collected in my youth, reminders of my favorite players. When I looked at them I could remember the heroics and surprises I had witnessed. Judith became my unlikely star, surviving what had seemed like a fatal condition.

After she left and Annie died, I moved on to my next rotation, in the emergency department. The ER, as we called it then, was completely different from ward medicine. It was a chaotic, smelly, noisy, crowded place, and I loved it. All day and all night, people of all kinds passed through the ER doors, and it did not matter if they had money or not. Bankers lay next to thieves, professors next to uneducated, homeless schizophrenics, and only the severity of the illness determined how long a person would wait to see a doctor. Some patients spoke Spanish and told stories of how they worked now as roofers or vegetable pickers or ranchers, and about their families back in Mexico. Others spoke Navajo and lived on the reservation, where they herded sheep and went to medicine men first when they got sick. The stories were endless and fascinating. An old man who fell from his roof while trying to fix his swamp cooler had once been a famous artist; he sketched staff and patients as he waited for us to sew up his forehead. A police officer fell off his motorcycle chasing a man who had robbed a convenience store; he cried when we stuck an IV into his arm. Then the robber of the convenience store arrived with a bullet in his stomach, surrounded by three other policemen, and the two patients looked at each other from across the room before we took the robber to the operating room for surgery.

Every day differed from the one before. One day might present a cluster of depressed people who had overdosed on medications; another day might feature patients with chest pains and heart attacks. I would wonder how the patients from one day might feel about their lives if given a moment to experience the lives of the patients from another day.

The emergency department demanded concentration and commitment. Sometimes if you worked fast, you could shock someone's heart back to life or pass a tube into the trachea and push air into the lungs. You could save a life in a few seconds and count up the saves and tubes at the end of the week like baskets of apples at harvest. You would lose track of time. Days and nights blended together until you suddenly felt hungry or exhausted and looked at your watch and realized that most people were home asleep. And you'd feel proud to be awake and working and keeping the department alive.

If Carl had worked in a hospital, he probably would have ended up in the emergency department, caring for the alcoholics, homeless men, prostitutes, and drug addicts who came there for all their care and often ended up on stretchers in the hallways watching the constant flow of ambulances, nurses, and doctors. Carl would not have worried about the effect of the nights and weekends on his personal life because his work and his personal life were inseparable.

Toward the end of the month, Judith returned. She was vomiting blood. Her face was pale and there was blood on her lips.

"Hello, Judith," I said. "Have you been drinking?"

She looked at the ground and then at the basin with dark clots of blood in it. "Yes," she said.

"OK," I said. "We'll have to admit you again and give you a blood transfusion and hope the bleeding stops." I called the admitting team, and the resident passed me to Rick because she was a bounce back. She had been on Rick's team and now had returned, so he had to take her back even though this was not his admitting day.

"Rick," I said, "Judith is back. Sorry. She's bleeding, and she's been drinking again."

"I told you this would happen. We should have let her die. This is why I hate internal medicine, why I'm going to switch into emergency medicine. Because internal medicine patients never get better. They just keep coming back until they die. At least in the ER you can see them and send them to someone else who has to see them every day."

"Sorry, Rick," I said.

I felt sad for her and sorry for embarrassing her with the question about drinking, but I was angry that all my work to keep her alive might be wasted, that she didn't care enough to stop. And I was upset that Rick had been right.

Several hours later a nurse wheeled her away to the intensive care unit. As I waved good-bye, I wondered what she was going to have to endure now. She waved back at me, a hopeful smile on her face, as if she were leaving on a train at the beginning of a long journey.

Chapter Twenty-one

MY THOUGHTS ABOUT MY DAYS AS A MEDICAL STUDENT and intern were interrupted when the phone rang.

It was Laura.

"Hi," she said. "I just wanted to see how you were doing."

"I'm . . . I'm OK," I said. "Actually, I'm a wreck. A guy came by and wanted to buy our house."

"Our house?"

"Yes."

"Did you already put it on the market?"

"No," I said.

"Then why would he come over to try to buy it?"

"I don't know," I said. "I guess someone saw you moving out. One of the neighbors called him. Some friend of his."

"Vultures, that's what they are," she said.

"So I guess that was my crisis for today," I said.

"Well, I talked to the kids. I called them at camp, and they sounded fine."

"Fine? Aren't they upset?"

"No, they seemed OK. Lots of activities, horseback riding, basketball."

"Well, that's nice," I said.

"I told them you were going to Mexico, and they were very excited," she said.

"Really?"

"Yes, well, you've told them so many stories about it over the years.

They know most of the characters. And they know how important it is to you."

"Well, that's interesting," I said. "I didn't realize it had such an impact upon them."

"Oh, it's had an impact upon all of us. Even me."

"Really?"

"Sure, don't you remember?"

"Yes. Yes I do," I said.

"Well, sleep well." She said.

"Bye," I said.

When I hung up, I thought about what she had said. Maybe she was just trying to be nice. But it made me stop and consider, and I thought back to when we first met and when I took her with me the last time I went back to Mexico.

We first met at a hot spring. In a hot spring in the mountains of New Mexico, you notice things: the feel of sand and pumice against your legs and back as you sit in the warm pool, the steam drifting up out of the clear water into your nostrils and eyes, the cooling breeze across your forehead and chest, the birds in the pines calling, answering, calling, answering. You notice a red pickup far away down the mountain in the parking lot; a small pine tree sticking out of the back of the pickup; the emergence of two women from the truck—one slim with light brown hair, and the other stooped, darker, older; and their steady progress along the trail until they reach the pool and stand there staring at us, my brother Ron and me. We smiled up at them before staring out at the mountains again to allow them privacy to disrobe.

But I watched as the younger one removed her jeans and then her shirt and folded them neatly before stuffing them in a crevice in the rocks. And then she removed her underwear, exposing a lithe, pale-skinned body, which she quickly hid beneath the water, leaving only her face exposed, the crimson lips and gray-green eyes, thick brown eyebrows, and long straight chestnut hair.

"Ooh, it's hot," she said.

And then the older woman got in and spoke. "I've always wanted to come here, but I didn't want to come by myself. My daughters would never let me go with them."

They pretended they were alone now, stopped conversing, closed their eyes, and then opened them and stared across the valley at the granite rock face and the forest. The hot spring had a long tradition of serving as a place of healing and contemplation, where each person could feel at peace and serene. They seemed to be seeking such a peaceful contemplative state.

After fifteen minutes, they were done. As she stepped from the pool and dressed, I noticed the curve of her back, the way she held her shoulders, her small breasts, the ampleness of her hips.

"Your underwear just fell into the mud," I said.

"Oh. Oh, thank you," she said and finally met my eyes with a shy smile. She picked up the underwear and gracefully toweled off her legs and feet.

We met them again in the parking lot.

"Hi," I said. "Is that your Christmas tree?"

"Yes. Yes it is. We cut it down today. That's why we were so filthy and dusty."

She pronounced her words crisply and rapidly.

"Are you from here?" I said.

"Well, I'm actually visiting my parents in Santa Fe, but I work in New York City. I'm here for the holidays."

"What do you do in the city?"

"I am an assistant to the editor of a woman's magazine, *Savvy Magazine*."

"Wow, so you get to meet writers and celebrities. I think I've seen it at the bookstore."

"Yes, it is at the bookstores and in grocery stores. We've been publishing for three years. Our target audience is professional women, but we've been picking up a broader feminist audience lately."

"You don't talk like a New Mexican," I said.

"Well, I was born here, spent my wonder years here, but I attended college in the East, at Wesleyan."

"I almost went there," I said. "I grew up near Boston, but I decided to go west to Stanford."

"Stanford, that's a wonderful school."

By now the other woman had produced a jug of wine and four glasses. "Hi, I'm Molly," she said. "And this is my niece, Laura. Would you like some wine?"

"Yes," I said. "I'm David, and this is my brother Ron, out visiting from Ohio."

"And David, where do you live?" asked Molly as she passed me a glass of red wine.

"In Albuquerque. I work at the University of New Mexico."

"What do you do there?" asked Molly.

"I'm a doctor. I work in the ER," I said.

"Very nice," said Molly as we sipped our wine. "Laura, maybe you might want to invite David and his brother up to Santa Fe?"

Laura looked at me and smiled. "I'll give you my number in Santa Fe," she said. "Perhaps if you want, you could call me." She wrote her name and number on a torn piece of napkin and handed it to me. I clutched it in my palm like a jewel as I walked back to my car.

The red pickup backed out onto the road, and the two women disappeared in a cloud of dust. My brother looked at me and smiled. "When you gonna call her?" he asked.

"I don't know," I said.

"If you don't, I will," he said.

I met her family at our first date a week later. We were going for a hike and then dinner. Her father extended a pink, fleshy hand in greeting and seemed relieved that I worked and, even better, was a physician. Though it was late morning, he offered me a glass of wine like what he was drinking. "Heck, it's almost lunchtime," he said. "Where are you going for dinner?"

When I told him, he said, "Get the rack of lamb, and here, take this bottle of wine. It's better than anything they have. Just ask them to open it." And he handed me a bottle of cabernet sauvignon.

Laura's mother hugged me.

"We're so happy to meet you," she said. "Laura has told us all about you. Perhaps after dinner, if you want some private time together, you could go to Laura's grandmother's apartment. She is out of town."

"Thanks," I said as Laura blushed.

We hiked in the mountains that day. Laura walked too fast up the hills and got out of breath.

"I'm not used to the mountains," she said.

"You should slow down," I said.

"No, I walk fast and talk fast," she said.

Later we went to the restaurant and both ordered the rack of lamb.

"Your parents are . . . nice," I said.

"They like you," she said.

"But they don't know me," I said.

"Well, I guess they know you enough. You made a good impression." Her eyes sparkled in the candlelight, and her hair glittered gold.

"So, I'm from the East living in the West, and you're from the West living in the East. I guess we've both come to about the same point in our evolution," I said.

"I like the East," she said. "People read books and talk about them and discuss ideas."

"Yes, but you lose touch with the environment. You're indoors and it's dark and cold and rainy. And in the summer, the beaches are all crowded or private."

"Well, in New Mexico you may find sand, but you won't find beaches. So what kind of doctor are you?"

"Emergency medicine," I said.

"Is that a specialty, or are you going to do something else?"

"It's a specialty now. It used to be different. Surgeons or internists would work in emergency departments while they started their practices, but now it is a specialty. I like it because it's always exciting, and you can save lives. But I think I'd like to work in a developing country at some point. I'd feel more useful. I did it in Mexico, before medical school, and I really felt like I made a difference. Of course, they don't pay very much, so I'd still have to work in the United States some of the time. What about you? Do you like New York?"

"It's fun. And New York is fascinating. The art galleries and the writers. I'd love to have a big house and host gatherings of writers and be part of their conversations," she said. "But New Mexico is in my blood. I think I'll come back eventually."

"They're all so pretentious, the writers and intellectuals. All they want to do is talk and talk. They'd rather describe a beautiful sunset than go outside and watch it," I said, and we laughed.

After dinner she took me to her grandmother's apartment because it was late and I'd had two glasses of wine. The apartment was cold.

"My grandmother must have turned down the heat," Laura said as we shivered.

We kissed after she showed me around the apartment. She stood at the doorway, and the kiss lingered magically. And then she came back inside. "Would you like me to stay?" she asked.

"Sure," I said, my voice shaking.

We made tea and sipped slowly, quietly.

"Do you live by yourself?" she asked.

"I just bought a house, and I got a roommate to help pay the mortgage," I said. "What about you?"

"I have an apartment in the city. It's a one bedroom on the ground floor, and the ceiling has a crack in it that looks like South America."

We both wanted to know if there were current boyfriends or girlfriends in our lives. It was a delicate question that could have caused the magic of the evening to evaporate; yet we felt ourselves drawn insistently toward it.

Finally she asked, "Are you involved with anyone?"

"Uh, well, no. I had a girlfriend but we broke up five months ago," I said.

"Isn't that amazing," she said. "I broke up with my boyfriend six months ago."

As the warmth of the tea dissipated, I began to shake. The apartment was uncomfortably cold, with just enough heat to keep the pipes from freezing.

"We could get into bed and warm up," she said.

"Well, sure, OK," I said, and we got under the heavy covers, still in our clothes, our teeth chattering, holding each other, her hand rubbing my neck.

The room smelled of dried lavender and talcum powder, which sat in bottles on a walnut bedside table. A Japanese kimono hung from a hook on the closet, and red and green Japanese slippers lay on the floor next to the kimono. Pictures of children and grandchildren spread out across the bureau.

She asked me about my family.

"My parents grew up in the same small city just outside Boston. It was where their parents settled after coming across the ocean from Russia in the early 1900s. My grandfather hid in a pickle barrel on a boat from Russia," I said.

"A pickle barrel?" she said.

"A *kosher* pickle barrel."

"Oh, are you Jewish?" she asked.

"Yes," I said.

"Wesleyan had lots of Jewish students. They were the smart ones."

"Well, Jewish parents put education above almost everything else.

My parents didn't want me to play football because I might injure my brains."

"What did they think of non-Jewish girls?"

"Shiksas, they called them. There were nice Jewish girls, and there were shiksas. The shiksas were usually blond, blue eyed, long legged, thin, and small nosed. Jewish girls were dark, smart, big breasted, and big nosed."

"Would I be considered a shiksa?"

"Oh yes, you would definitely be considered a shiksa. You'd be a prototype except that you went to Wesleyan and work in New York City. But even so, you would qualify."

"How do you feel about shiksas?" she asked.

"Well, I've hardly even gone out with Jewish girls. So I guess you could say I like them. Jewish girls get too focused on the idea that I am a doctor; it seems to overwhelm everything else. But I didn't become a doctor to create an estate for a Jewish princess. I want to be free to take care of people anywhere in the world no matter how poor they are. I don't want to worry about car payments, house payments, private school tuition, and a maid. I just want to be able to be with someone who wants me for who I am, and not what I can get for them."

Laura hugged me, and I kissed her. She laughed nervously.

"You're a good kisser," she said.

"So are you," I said.

As we rubbed against each other through our clothes, we gradually became familiar with our bodies under the clothes. We touched a shoulder, an arm, and a thigh. Gradually our clothes came off. First the sweater and the skirt, then the pants, and finally the underwear.

We lay there skin to skin under the heavy quilt trembling from the cold and the excitement.

"Do you want . . . ?" I asked.

"Yes. Yes, I do," she said. "But only if you do." And she kissed me and let her hair fall over my face. I felt her body dance over mine as she kissed me. We held each other for a while and then kissed again as our hands wandered and touched every hidden place, and then we stopped again, feeling each other. We held each other the entire night and finally made love at dawn.

In the morning I brought her back to her house. Her dad was in the kitchen drinking coffee.

"I guess you're still here," he said. "Would you like some coffee?"

"Yes, thanks," I said.

Six months later Laura moved out from New York to be with me, and we got married four months after that. After we married we could have gone anywhere for our honeymoon—China, Nepal, Peru, or Tahiti—anywhere in the world. Her father had offered this as his gift to us.

"Mexico, I'd like to go back to Mexico," I said. "It will give us time to plan our life. We can stay on the beach in San Blas, and I can show you the clinic where I worked, and you can meet the people there."

"What about Florence, Italy? We could go to the museums and eat at the four-star restaurants and then go to Paris."

"No, it's too formal. Too many tourists, too much money. Even though your dad is paying, I'd feel uncomfortable. We'll be alone in Mexico. Just the two of us. We'll find places. Beautiful places, just for us."

"OK," she said. And there was a sigh of resignation as Florence evaporated to be replaced by Mexico. We made our plans, took a plane down, and began our honeymoon in Mexico.

We found a hotel on the beach for several days and took a boat up a river to see herons and pelicans. Our room had a fan that moved the warm, humid air around, and we drifted on the starched sheets between sleeping and dreaming, embracing, kissing, making love. We'd get up to find a restaurant, walk to the beach, and float in the waves. Laura wore a straw hat, and even with sunscreen, her pale skin turned red.

"Let's leave the beach," I said. "Let's go to the village. It's only four hours away."

"Are you sure?" she asked. "Don't go just because of my sunburn."

"No, I want to go. I want you to see it. I want you to know me through it."

"OK. I could probably use a break from the beach."

We arrived at the village in our rented VW Beetle. I parked outside Ricardo and Rosa's house. Eight years had passed since I had worked at the clinic. I had completed medical school and residency, and now I was a faculty member at a medical school. I was a different person, and I wondered about our reception as we appeared now without warning after these years of silence. The entryway to the house had changed, and now a small storefront protruded into the sidewalk. Rosa stared from behind the counter, trying to figure out who had parked a car in front of her house. As I stepped out from the car, a great smile of recognition came over her face.

"David, David," she said, and she opened the gate and hurried forward, grabbing my hand and then embracing me.

"Mucho gusto," I said.

"Qué David," she said. "So much time. But I knew you would come back."

And then Laura stepped out from the other door. Rosa nodded and looked to me for an introduction.

"This is my wife, Laura," I said.

"¿Su esposa?" she asked. Your wife? "I did not know you were married."

I showed her our rings. She examined them and remarked, "How beautiful." And then she called to Ricardo inside the house.

"Hola, David," he said, grasping my hand. And then, shaking Laura's hand, he asked, "Is it true? Is this your wife?"

"Yes," I said. "This is Laura."

"Mucho gusto," he said. "Ricardo, at your command." And then he added after a short pause, "Is she pregnant yet?"

"Pregnant? Well, I don't think so," I said.

Laura and I had talked about children and had decided that we would let nature take its course. But we were not ready to discuss it in public.

"Good, then you can sleep in our matrimonial bed. It has brought us six children, and it will bring you a child also," he said and showed me the bed, a heavy wooden box. Wedding pictures of the family and a crucifix of Jesus hung on the wall at the head of the bed.

"Oh, but where will you sleep?" I said. I did not want to displace them, and I had never slept beneath a crucifix.

But he insisted. "There are cots; we will be fine. This will be our wedding gift to you."

I translated to Laura, and her face blushed a deep red. Ricardo laughed, and Rosa chided him for laughing and embarrassing Laura. Then we carried our suitcases into the house. I had forgotten the immediate contrast of the dark, cool adobe and the oppressive heat of the street. Our eyes gradually adjusted to the pastel pink walls. We sat down at the kitchen table and Rosa scooped water from an earthen jug with a gourd.

"This water has been boiled," she said to reassure us.

"Gracias," I said as I drank thirstily. The water dribbled from my lips.

"Gracias," said Laura.

"Very red, her face," commented Ricardo.

"Very pretty," said Rosa.

I told them about medical school, the years as an intern and resident, the studying and tests, the relentless work hours, and the sick who would not survive.

"How terrible," he said. "Why couldn't you cure them?"

"Sometimes they would not get better," I said. "Even with all of our medicine and antibiotics."

"Yes, sometimes it is the will of God," he said. "But don Carlos does not believe in that. He does not believe in the will of God."

The clinic walls lay ten feet away across the alley. I was tempted to leave Ricardo and Laura and look at the clinic. It drew me powerfully, and I wondered if Carl was there.

"How are your children?" I asked.

"Oh, they are all studying. Tomás is at the university. He is studying commerce. Remember Paulo, who loved animals? He is studying to be a veterinarian. The others are in secondary school. Only Marta is still here with us." A little girl of eight or nine suddenly ran and buried her face in her mother's arms.

"She's embarrassed," said Rosa.

"Perhaps you would like to visit the clinic," said Ricardo.

"Well, yes, I was thinking of showing it to Laura."

"Of course," said Ricardo.

"Con permiso." I asked to take leave.

"Como no," said Ricardo.

"We'll be back in a little while," I said.

Laura grabbed my hand as we walked over to the clinic. She followed willingly, innocently, and I knew I shouldn't be doing it, taking her there on our honeymoon, but I was irresistibly drawn back. I recognized the old pictures and posters still on the waiting room wall and the long hard bench now empty. No patients were waiting, and the clinic was dark. I realized it was the midday lunch break and everyone—doctors, patients, and assistants—had gone. As I walked through the rooms, I inhaled the smells of powdered medicine and dust. I felt my body reacting as if to a drug. The waves of excitement, fear, power, and wonder surged over me. The dental chair, its green plastic peeling off, remained exactly where I remembered it. Perhaps Laura noticed my reaction.

"Are you OK?" she asked.

"Yes, it's just kind of overwhelming to be back here. I feel a little dizzy," I said.

"Why?" she asked.

"I don't know. It's like seeing someone you thought was dead."

"Let's go out into the backyard," Laura said, and she led me out into the portal where the patients would sometimes stay. I remembered how Demetrio stayed out there while we treated his burn. And Carl would sometimes be out there in the loft. As we walked into the courtyard, a woman eating rice and beans jumped to her feet.

"Is there something I can do for you?"

"I am David. I used to work here in the clinic eight years ago. Now I am a doctor in New Mexico," I said and shook her hand.

"Yes, I have heard about you. But they said you would not come back again. My name is Maria Nuñez," she said. "I am the assistant for the clinic."

"Yes, well it has been a long time, but here I am with my wife, Laura," I said.

Maria Nuñez shook Laura's hand.

"I was wondering about Carl, Gabriel, Luis, and Deanna. Are any of them here?"

"Well, Gabriel is taking his lunch. Deanna is in the United States. I do not know what she is doing there. And Luis is studying in the United States. He is studying to be a dental technician. Carl is resting up in the loft. Perhaps he will see you later."

And then I heard the sound of boxes moving and steps on the wood. Legs emerged down the ladder until finally his face was visible, and he stood there just as I had remembered him. His hair and beard now sprouted patches of gray, and he wore dusty blue jeans and a T-shirt that said *Venceremos*. We shall conquer. Even his politics were the same. He took a few steps toward me before stopping to stare at Laura.

"So you've come back to help us at the clinic. We've been waiting for you. We can certainly use the help." And then he extended his hand to Laura.

"Carl Wilson," he said. "Welcome to La Clínica. Did I overhear David say that you are his new wife?"

"Yes," said Laura.

"Well, you are quite welcome here. I always thought David had a very keen eye for beauty, and now you have confirmed that."

"Thank you," she said.

And then he came over to me. "Congratulations," he said, and he pulled me close with a one-armed hug and a pat on the back. "You should have written. We wondered what had happened to you."

"I'm sorry. I was so busy with medical school and residency," I muttered.

"Are you still in medical school?" he asked.

"No. I graduated and then specialized in emergency medicine. Now I'm on the faculty at the University of New Mexico."

"Very impressive. You could teach us a lot if you could stay a few weeks."

"Yes, I know, but we're just here on our honeymoon. I wanted to show Laura the clinic. We're only staying here with Ricardo and Rosa until tomorrow. I'll be back for a longer visit soon," I said.

"Don't wait too long. We are struggling with the government. They are trying to decide whether to put a government clinic here to compete with us. But the people of the village are very loyal. And Gabriel has become a health *promotor*. He works here with me and takes over when I go back to the United States. We have visitors from all over the world who want to replicate what we have done."

"It sounds wonderful," I said.

A boy of about fourteen walked up to us. He limped and had a crutch in his left hand. "This is Marcelo," said Carl. "He has a weak left side, perhaps from meningitis or polio. We have a program now for disabled children and adults to help them learn skills to care for themselves and support themselves. Marcelo is helping us here at the clinic."

Marcelo smiled at us and shook my hand and then Laura's hand.

"Marcelo would have died without the program," Carl said.

"I think I'll show Laura the village," I said.

"Nice to meet you," Carl said to Laura, and then to me he said, "We really could use your help."

Laura and I walked the streets of the village. Some people stared at us, and I wondered if I recognized a child I had treated, now grown into a teenager, or a man with tuberculosis who had come to me for streptomycin injections. I showed Laura the river and the swimming hole. Children were swimming in bathing suits. "Eight years ago everyone swam naked," I said. "So what do you think?"

"I don't know. It's really hot and dusty here, but I can see why you like it."

We returned to Ricardo and Rosa's house. They had slaughtered a chicken, and it cooked over the fire next to boiling beans. "We are so happy you remembered us," said Rosa.

"Of course," said Ricardo. "He is part of our family."

"Thank you," I said.

I savored every bite of food and the shadows that danced across the walls.

That night as Laura and I lay in the matrimonial bed under the crucifix, I reminded her of the history of the bed.

"Sure," she said. "I can't think of a better place." And she came to me enveloped in a sheet as lizards scampered across the walls, chasing insects.

We talked of our future life together, of travel to exotic lands, of children, of sharing adventures, of uncertainty and risk.

"I'm not afraid of anything but boredom," she said.

"OK," I said. And I told her about the chaos in the emergency department when someone was dying in front of your eyes, and how I wanted to be there at that moment. "It's never boring," I said.

She smiled and pulled me toward her.

I told her about Carl and the staff at the clinic, how they attracted people like a magnet, mesmerizing, hypnotizing all of us who came under their spell.

"You can come back sometime, but you're mine now," she said and smothered me in kisses. "I can be wild."

From across the alley, the clinic called for me in the night with lights and voices, a crying baby. I lay waiting for the fists to pound at the door and voices to call my name, "David, David, por favor." But the lights went out and the moment passed. I heard every noise that night and wanted to remember everything.

And that night, as Ricardo predicted, a child was conceived in the matrimonial bed.

Chapter Twenty-two

I HAD NIGHTMARES ABOUT MY HOUSE: IT HAD BEEN BOUGHT by the television newsman and converted to a studio with actors and actresses. I woke up in the dark wondering where I was. At 2:30 a.m., the night still stretched far ahead, and I had to confront it all alone. By morning, I was happy to go to work just to be able to get out of the house.

I had a full day of evaluations with faculty scheduled, and I expected them to keep my mind focused. Each hour another faculty member knocked on my door and tentatively took a seat. It surprised me sometimes to think that these adults in their thirties, forties, and fifties could act like schoolchildren about to receive their report cards. They would dwell on every word, look for hidden meanings, argue about a criticism, cry, become angry, have tears of joy, or sigh with relief at the end.

Rick was my last appointment of the day. I told him some of the criticisms from the nurses and what he needed to do to change their opinions. Even after all the years, the reversal of authority from our previous relationship, when he was the resident and I was the intern, still felt awkward.

"I'll meet with them," he said. "I don't like to get bad grades."

"It's not exactly a bad grade. You're a wonderful researcher and a great teacher, but this is an opportunity for improvement. Maybe we need to do a better job of aligning incentives."

"Sounds like you've been reading those management books," he said. "You've got the lingo down."

Rick walked over to the window of my office and looked across the street to the drab, brown buildings that made up the undergraduate campus. "You can look right into the dormitories," he said. "The girls' dormitory."

"No, you can't," I said. "Anyway, that building is the dining hall."

"Yeh—huh," Rick hooted. "I really got you with that one. Your face turned red."

"I've got to get back to work," I said.

"You know, all this work you do—all the memos, all the meetings, all of the letters to unhappy patients who complain about waiting too long, all the e-mails to hospital administrators about why we aren't collecting enough money or why we should have more nurses or why someone died in the waiting room after sitting for eight hours—everyone will forget that you did that stuff the day after you leave. And a few days later, they'll forget you were even chairman, and a few days after that, they'll forget you were even here. They will say, 'Oh yeah, that was when that other guy—what was his name?—was chairman.' I've watched what happens when people leave. It's like they bring in a fresh coat of paint, and nothing's left from before."

"Well, at least the patients will remember. And the residents; they'll remember we were here."

"Hell, our patients can't even remember to take their medicines. Do you think they will remember you?"

"Well, the ones we take care of over the years. They'll remember."

"So you've entrusted your place in history to the memory of our chronic seizure patients, the drunks, and the sicklers. To Clayton Jones, Mary Joe, and Pedro Nieto. None of them will be around very long. If those are your historians, you might as well make it all up. The only way people remember you is if you are a mass murderer. No, nothing that any of us has done in the ER will matter to anyone after we leave this place."

"Well, it will matter to me," I said.

"OK, when you and I retire we'll sit down with a few glasses of beer, and then we'll see how much it will all matter to either of us," he said.

"Rick, I never realized you were such a cynic," I said.

"I'm a realist. I know what motivates people. It's money, sex, and power—not necessarily in that order. Doing good things is not even on the list except maybe for priests, and we know that for them, young boys are a lot higher on the list. I would never trust a do-gooder, because I'd know that his true intentions and motivations were hidden."

"So what motivates you?" I asked.

"Well, these days, breaking the boredom is enough. That's what keeps me going down to the ER. But I'm just biding my time until retirement, trying to pay the bills, fly my model planes, and have time with my wife. You know we've been married thirty years."

"That's great," I said.

"Sorry," he said. "I didn't mean to bring that up again."

"It's OK; you've pretty much trashed everything else in my life," I said.

Rick came over and put his arms around me. We hugged.

It was an odd moment, feeling his big hands on my back, the tangle of his beard on my forehead, the smell of his pipe tobacco, after twenty years of rounds in the ER, faculty meetings, and resident conferences. So many times we had turned to each other at the end of a shift, entrusting to one another a sick baby or an injured friend. So many times we had shared a loss, laughed at an absurdity, denounced our bosses as incompetent, and wondered how we could continue.

Day after day for twenty years, we had first created a residency, then a department bit by bit from nothing. Day after day we had helped each other with our papers, argued about problems, worked on our promotions to associate professor, then professor. And now this hug.

Rick released me, and we stepped apart.

"Are you OK?" he asked.

"I guess so," I said.

"It's weird, all the people who split up. I never thought it would be you," he said.

"Neither did I," I said. "She said it isn't about me. That it is just something she has to do, that she still loves me, but she needs to live apart."

"Well, I think it's something women are reading about, and encouraging each other to do, to prove they are equal to men. In the days when everyone struggled to survive, and the men worked in the fields all day while the women cooked and brought up the kids, this wouldn't have happened. But now, people split up for no reason. I mean, you're not a drunk or drug addict; you're not gambling away money. There's no girlfriend or boyfriend. She even says she still loves you. And you have two kids and a nice house. It makes no sense at all," he said.

"I guess I could have been more romantic. We could have gone out on dates. I could have bought her flowers and clothes. But my head was always full of errands to do, papers to write, homework to do with the kids. She wanted excitement, and I just wanted to rest. She'd fall asleep before I went to bed. But I thought we were OK. I didn't know she was unhappy. I just thought we were all tired from working so hard," I said.

"Yeah, I guess we don't know what they're thinking when they're home alone all night, and we're up all night working in the ER. Then we come home and sleep during the day and can't talk because we're so wiped out. It's just a big blur for us, but it isn't the same for them," he said. "They have too much time alone. We need the extended families where Grandma and Grandpa are around to keep an eye on things. But we're all spread out all over the country. Aren't your parents back East?"

"Yeah, they're in Boston and still married. They can't understand it."

"Well, the strangest thing I've noticed is that some people fight and hate each other, but they stay together. Other people get along and seem good together, but they break up. It's sort of like our patients in the ER. You'll see someone who looks old and weak and ready to die, and that will be the one who fights on and leaves the hospital. And others look fine, healthy and go just like that, right before your eyes as you're telling them that they're gonna be OK. I suppose if you were religious, you'd say that it was God deciding. And when it's your time, then it's your time."

"Well, if that's the case, how do you know whether to fight it? If it's all determined, why not just give up?"

"'Cause maybe I'm wrong, and it isn't fated. Do you want to take that chance?" Rick laughed and took out his pipe. "I hardly smoke this thing anymore. But I like to hold it and think about smoking it," he said.

The smell of tobacco was still strong as he held the pipe. It conjured up the many meetings over the years when he had puffed at the pipe, considering an idea or how to fix one of our research studies. But with the bans on indoor smoking, he had pretty much abandoned the pipe. Its presence now was like a reunion with an old friend whose face and body reminded you of the passage of time and whose voice kindled memories that had long been irretrievable. An old friend who held memories that spiraled and drifted away like smoke.

The daylight was fading as I looked out across the campus. The strange twists of fate Rick had brought up reminded me of how the Mexican clinic and the people I met there kept reappearing in my life long after I had left. I wondered if there was a puppeteer pulling invisible strings, and in my most paranoid moments, I related it all to Carl and his sphere of influence. Perhaps our encounters were coincidence, or perhaps they were the natural outcomes based upon our shared interests. As I recalled each incident that had occurred over the years, I was more determined than ever to go back to the village, to find the thread that connected us. It had to be there. How else could I explain the chance meeting with Luis in San Francisco after my visit to the village? Neither of us should have been there, and yet there we were.

I was walking up a hill in San Francisco, looking for a hotel where I was to attend a conference, and Luis spotted me. I heard someone shout my name, "David, David!" I looked around and saw a young man running toward me. "It's me—Luis."

"Luis?" I said. I recognized his exuberant, bright eyes, now surrounded by beefier jowls and a moustache, but he was still the Luis I knew from the clinic. "Luis? What are you doing here?"

"I live in California now," he said. "This is my wife." He pointed at a breathless woman who had hurried up behind him as he sprinted toward me. "This is my wife, Julia." The woman beamed at me as I shook her hand. She had very light skin and long black hair, and her cheeks burned red as she tried to think of something to say.

"Mucho gusto," I said.

"Thanks," she said. "I don't know much Spanish."

"So, Luis," I said. "What are you doing here? And how did you recognize me?"

"I live here. I'm a dental assistant. I saw you walking, and I knew it was you."

"Well, that's amazing. Because I don't live here. I'm just visiting. I live in New Mexico with my wife. How's the clinic? And Carl? Have you spoken to him lately?" I asked without considering the passage of years or the impact of his marriage upon his feelings.

"Well, Carl doesn't talk to me. He doesn't like me to stay up here. He wants me to come back and work in the clinic, but I don't want to, and Julia doesn't want to, either." Julia nodded to emphasize her resolve.

"I don't like the place," she said. "It isn't safe, and it's not a good place for Luis except for visiting his parents. And Carl is sort of strange," she added.

"Yes," I said.

"It's changing," said Luis. "It's not the same. Even Carl is not there so much anymore. So we are happy to be here."

"Well, good. You seem happy," I said, though I could sense a tinge of sadness and wistfulness in his eyes.

"Yes, I'm very happy here. I have a nice job. And Julia does too. I work at the French Hospital Dental Clinic. We have a little house in the Mission. You should visit us. Julia is a great cook."

He beamed at her and squeezed her hand. Her cheeks flushed red again, and he kissed them and laughed. "I call her my little tomato," he said.

We talked about old friends for a while. Deanna and Tony had separated after living together for six years. She had gone back to the village. "I think Tony is *poco loco*," he said. A little crazy.

Luis said that the drugs were worse than ever, with more guns and soldiers. Almost every month someone was getting shot or arrested. The clinic had almost been closed, but Carl had gone to Mexico City for a special meeting with the president, and it remained open. The government had opened its own clinic in town with a Mexican doctor.

"I was there last year, but you know more than I do," I said.

"I find out from the other volunteers and my family too. You know, some of the volunteers live here in San Francisco. But Carl is so busy with his new projects. He's traveling all over the world," he said.

"I'm sure he would want to hear from you," I said. But I wondered how Carl felt about Luis now, eight years later. Luis was no longer young, no longer a teenager, no longer handsome, no longer dependent on Carl or his money. I wondered what happened to Luis and all the other Luises when they grew up.

"What about you?" he asked.

"Well, I just had my first child, a girl," I said. "That's why my wife is not here with me. She's home with the baby. We hardly ever get to sleep through the night anymore. And I work in an emergency room in Albuquerque. I'm on the faculty at the university. That's about all there's time for now."

Luis gave me a wink like he used to when he wanted me to know that he understood a private joke that was hidden from others. The wink made me stop and wonder what he thought I might be doing. He was used to concealment and hidden meanings.

"Ay, David, you work too much," he said.

"Como no," I said, because he was right. There always seemed to be more to do than the time I had to do it. One more patient, one more article, and one more lecture.

"Quién sabe," he said, to complete our own internal joke. I smiled to acknowledge the memory of who we were when we had last been together and his subtle question of who I was now.

"Como no," I repeated.

There wasn't much else to say. I told him I'd write, and he thanked me. "We'll have dinner together," I said. He seemed small and lost as he retreated down the road with his wife. He didn't belong in San Francisco amid the tall concrete buildings. But the idea of Luis married and independent and working as a dental assistant also satisfied me. After all the years that I wondered about the relationship between Carl and Luis, I could finally see a resolution, an acceptable end, with Luis happy, productive, and married, and Carl off on new campaigns for social justice. Life seemed to have worked out for both of them, and I didn't want to think more about how or why. Instead, I thought about his wink. I was amazed at the coincidence of our meeting, the huge odds against it having happened. I delighted in the wonder of it all, the happy ending. Perhaps our universe was not so large, our paths not so disparate. And so we headed off in different directions.

As I walked back toward the hotel, a homeless man wearing a red Santa hat shoved a metal cup in front of me and asked for spare change for coffee. As I reached for a quarter, I knew that he would use it for cheap wine. But I still enjoyed the clink as it dropped into his cup, and his sincere "God bless you."

After replaying my encounter with Luis, I thought about how many other encounters had connected me again and again to the clinic. It was like a gravitational pull on planets and comets, which seem to sail around independently in the vastness of space yet are all connected to the force in the center. And at the center was Carl, with a shimmering light too bright and dangerous for our eyes to discern his true shape or nature.

Chapter Twenty-three

MY NEXT ENCOUNTER WITH THE CLINIC OCCURRED DURING a class that I took on international health. I had hoped it would give me perspective on my experience in Mexico, but later, as I watched the setting sun from my office, I realized that instead, the class had picked at my festering wound. As I contemplated my return to the village, I thought about one particular meeting. The topic was identification of projects and approaches that had been successful all over the world. One evening the professor informed the class that we would be watching a movie about a clinic in Mexico.

"This movie is over twenty years old, but it is still the best example of a successful international development project," he said. "So many give out medicines, do a few surgeries, vaccinate a few children, but they make the people dependent on more outside help. The volunteers feel good because they see immediate results. But when they leave, nothing remains. Equipment wears out, and no one knows how to fix it. New problems appear, and no one has the skill or knowledge to solve them."

I sat on a cold metal desk chair with a foldable platform arm for note taking as I listened to the professor introduce the movie. The other attendees were doctors who, like me, taught at the medical school or worked in the hospital. We got together every month to talk and show slides. Our lectures were usually part travelogue, part epidemiology, and part shared fantasy of a different world and a different set of problems. As the professor slipped the cassette into the recorder and adjusted the television, I emptied my head of the day's patients to allow myself to experience whatever exotic place this might be.

"This project is different," the professor said as he adjusted the tape. "They provided medical care, but they also trained villagers, built a water system, a grain bank, and a sewage system. And they spent a tenth of what most experts estimate to be the minimum for such an ambitious undertaking." He pressed the play button, and the tape began to roll.

A man on muleback trotted down a dusty road past peeling adobe houses to the clinic with its La Clínica sign, and my heart sped up and skipped even before I knew why.

Luis appeared in the dental room pulling decayed teeth. The narrator explained how Luis had received training in the United States to provide basic dental services. By training local villagers, the skills would stay where they were needed. I watched as Luis anesthetized and pulled a tooth, calming the patient while he worked. The Luis of the movie was not only mature beyond his fifteen or sixteen years, but also spontaneous and exuberant as he pretended not to be aware of the camera. Loli, sweeping with his one arm, and Deanna, directing a group of children, became examples of the village sanitation program. Gabriel sat behind a table writing on index cards, unwilling to look up at the camera. I watched for telltale signs of Loli's craziness, a sudden leap into the air or an unexpected scream, but there were none. And Deanna, with her dark eyes and passionate smile, seemed small and lost among the children.

Carl discussed the philosophy of the clinic, comforted sick babies, and rode up to an isolated mountain farm on muleback with a bag of medicines. He described the new clean-water system built with the cooperation of all the villagers, though I knew it hadn't worked out as planned. Someone had thrown a dead goat into the well, polluting the water so that it was undrinkable. And the spigots from the well had been placed outside the homes of the wealthier villagers rather than being placed in the locations most convenient to everyone. Even Carl had compromised his principles.

Then he told a story of a village herbalist who had combined herbal remedies with scientific methods to bring the best of both worlds to his patients. Yet I knew that the herbalist could not remember which antibiotics to give, and that he had returned to his previous folk-medicine practice, abandoning the role that Carl had prepared for him.

Then the músico played a sad, heroic corrido about Valentín of the Sierra, who was shot and hanged for waging revolutionary war against the Spanish army. It was a solitary, isolated struggle against all odds, but even when Valentín lost, his spirit triumphed. The high, mournful sounds of the guitar and voice resonated with my memories, and I began to drift back to that time when Tony was making his movie.

When the tape finished, the professor stood up and asked if there were any questions or comments. "I was there," I said, "in 1972, as a volunteer before I went to medical school." Everyone looked over at me, and they seemed to study my face to see if they could place it in the movie. "I knew Carl Wilson," I added.

The professor nodded. "I have seen the success of projects like this as an extension of the personality of a charismatic leader. Does that fit your experience with Carl Wilson and this project?"

"Well, yes, without him it would never have lasted," I said. "But Carl has many layers, and so does the project."

"He must have had quite an influence on you."

I smiled and did not answer. It would have been easy and true to say yes. But *yes* did not convey my own doubts about the *nature* of the influence, an influence that covered me like a mineral residue after the slow evaporation of a storm—almost part of me, but separate. "He did," I said. "He taught me how much one person with determination can accomplish even against the odds, incredible odds. If you persevere and don't give up, you will draw others to you."

The professor thanked me, thanked everyone for coming, and announced the next session before the group dispersed. Except for me. I asked about the tape—where to buy one and whether I could borrow it.

"Of course," he said.

I took it home and watched it again. It was Carl's model of how he wanted the clinic to be, even if it wasn't completely true. I had carried the model with me, trying to stretch it or cut it to fit my life. I turned the sound off, which made the film a collage of places and people patched together to tell Carl's story. Without the narrator's words, the images of the film and my memories of the clinic could merge into something slightly out of focus but recognizable, familiar but strange, like a room in the dark of night.

Chapter Twenty-four

THE INTERNATIONAL-HEALTH CLASS ALSO LED ME BACK into contact with Carl. Some of the medical students whom I had met in the class wanted to invite Carl to be the medical school graduation speaker. He was becoming famous for his work at the clinic and the books he had written about it. The students were looking for a model of altruism. And since one student had been in the class when I admitted my past affiliation with the clinic, he asked me to call Carl and invite him to New Mexico.

I felt nervous about calling, because it had been so many years since we had worked closely together. Our most recent interaction at the clinic had been brief and awkward. What if he would not talk to me? What if I was just another face, another name from the past sufficiently faded from memory to exist only as background? But even more important, how did I feel about being a part of bringing him here as graduation speaker? I found myself driven by a sense of curiosity about who he now was and what he was doing, as if it might be somehow connected to me and my life. I wanted to talk to him.

But before I could talk to him, I had to find him. I started with the foundation staff, and they directed me to the home of a woman, a longtime supporter of Carl's work, who directed me to another home where he happened to be staying in preparation for a trip to Asia. The woman who answered the phone told me that Carl was famous now. His ideas were being used all over the world, even if the clinic was becoming a relic. Groups invited him for consultations and talks in England and Africa and South America. He had given keynote speeches and graduation addresses. She enumerated Carl's accomplishments and invitations as if his celebrity were now partially hers. It did not seem to matter that he was not a physician. In fact, he now proudly presented himself as a village health worker, a nonphysician, and a model for the parts of the world where physicians would not go. I thanked her for the update as she went to get him, and I wondered if he would sound different—aloof perhaps, or arrogant. But I also basked in the glow of his success, which seemed to validate my own ideas. If his years of toil and self-sacrifice were finally receiving recognition and support, maybe it could happen to me. Maybe my nights with the alcoholics, the homeless, the psychotics, and the bleeding gang members would also be honored, and I would be invited to address conferences in Asia. Yet even as I celebrated his success, I wondered how much the outside world knew about him and the clinic, and whether fame would expose his secrets. If I knew secrets after months with him, how much more must others know?

"Hello," Carl said when he answered my phone call.

"Hi, Carl," I said.

His voice materialized in stages, as if he were warming up his vocal cords. The words seemed to stumble as they became audible. I would have attributed it to a bad phone connection except that there was something familiar about the way his voice would gradually take form from indistinguishable sounds.

"Well, well. How are the aspiring physicians of New Mexico?" he asked.

"Oh, fine. They've suddenly discovered you and the clinic. They want you to be their graduation speaker. Any chance you might be able to visit us?"

"Well, I'm honored. Medical school is such an interesting blend of idealism and pragmatism. I'm afraid I might shock them or disappoint them. These days, I never know quite what I'll say or do until it sort of bursts out. But they all seem to like it, because they clap and pay me. They can listen, clap, and then go out and earn a million. Unfortunately the timing is bad. I'm about to leave for China and then to India. These international conferences are exhausting, but our message is reaching new receptive ears. It's very exciting."

"Well, so I guess you can't make it to the graduation. It's in two months."

"No."

"Maybe another time."

"Yes. There will be another time. Send me a letter. And if they can spare a small donation for the clinic, we always appreciate a little help; we need equipment, and the walls need painting. Perhaps you could be the speaker. I could authorize you to speak for me."

I thought about that. About standing in for Carl. Speaking for him. Representing him. I felt both proud and embarrassed. I wondered whether he thought of me as a disciple, carrying his message. Or was I merely useful? Another soldier in his army. Another tire to keep the vehicle rolling.

"No. No, I couldn't do that," I said.

"Of course you could. I could send you slides."

I remembered how he had convinced me years ago to read the books and become the doctor for the village. Now he was doing it again. Was he helping me to stretch, to become more than I thought I could be, or was he manipulating me for his own purposes?

This time I said no because I knew they wanted him, not me. Maybe a day would come when they might ask for me. I'd tell them about all the stories that spiraled out of the encounters between a doctor and a patient. And how each story provided a rare and unique moment of connection and exposure, a nakedness of body and spirit. And how, as doctors, they were guardians of that moment, that body, that spirit. Carl wouldn't tell that. He'd tell them to pick up every fallen body, dress every bleeding wound, and heal the world at all costs, because that was our responsibility to each other, our sacred mission. He'd tell them how one person could do this. I'd tell them that one person could not do it all. But one person could do a lot. And one person could influence others, and they could learn from each other, from their own stories. But they weren't asking for me, and I did not want to give Carl's speech.

I told the medical student that Carl couldn't come. He asked who might be a good alternative for a graduation speaker—someone with high ideals and ethics, a commitment to the poor, a sense of adventure, and a vision for the future. I think he picked an astronaut or a politician. But I know it wasn't Carl, and it wasn't me.

Chapter Twenty-five

A FEW MONTHS AFTER MY PHONE CONVERSATION WITH Carl, after a particularly frustrating resuscitation had failed, I ran into another person from our original group of La Clínica volunteers.

The unsuccessful resuscitation was not the nurse's fault. She had come from New York to fill in while we recruited new nurses to replace those who had recently left. Her name was Cindy, and she exuded confidence and toughness, from her body-builder biceps to her short black hair and crisp white scrubs. But she was a traveling nurse and should never have been in the trauma room by herself, where seconds wasted could mean death. Another nurse would have known immediately where to get the medicine, and how much to give. Instead, Cindy said that we didn't have any. I knew it wasn't her fault, and the patient, a man hit by a car as he was attempting to run across the highway to a bar, would probably have died anyway. But I walked out of the trauma room shaking my head and muttering about how much longer I could continue to work in this emergency department.

"Take a break," said Anna, a chunky, middle-aged clerk who had known me for years. She could see the frustration and disgust on my face. "We can manage for ten minutes."

So I rushed past the automatic doors out into the sunlight and realized that half the day was gone. Ambulances lined the parking lot, with names like Living Cross, Edgewood, Taos, and Superior. A display of sandals for sale drew a cluster of hospital visitors.

"Where are these sandals from?" asked a fat, bald man, wheezing as he spoke. I doubted he could take many steps in sandals before he would collapse and die.

"Mexico. We got them from Mexico. Poor, disabled village children make them, and we give the profits back to La Clínica where they live," said a thin, blond girl with a practiced sincerity. After answering the question, she stared out at the horizon while listening to a Walkman CD player.

"How much are these brown ones?" the man asked, pointing at sandals with brown straps on black rubber soles.

"Just twenty-five dollars," she said. I imagined the profits from these sandal sales being plowed back into my emergency department. Maybe then we could afford stretchers so that sick people didn't get put in chairs where they would collapse to the floor, or we could afford to have gowns so that the patients didn't have to wander the halls half naked, or we could afford to pay for enough nurses and doctors so that no one would have to wait the usual three or four hours to be seen and treated. As I watched the girl sell a pair of sandals, I recognized the style of sandal commonly worn in the village where I had worked in Mexico.

Then I saw a man in a brightly colored Guatemalan shirt join the blond girl; his deeply etched face wrinkled enthusiastically as he attempted to make change for the two twenty-dollar bills offered up as payment for the sandals. His wavy gray beard hung down from his lower lip in long swirls that twisted like rope and contrasted with his deeply tanned bald head. But his eyes looked familiar. "Tony?" I asked tentatively.

"David," he said and clasped his arms around me in a bear hug. "I thought I might find you here. This is my stepdaughter, Kora." He pointed to the blond girl once again absorbed in her music and staring off absently.

"Well, what are you doing here? How did you know you might find me? I've heard lots of strange rumors about you," I said in a burst of laughter as the words tumbled out.

"And I've heard them about you," he said. "Doctor, head of an emergency room, two kids, and a big, fancy house." He grinned back at me.

People around us were getting diverted from the sandals to our conversation. As I noticed our audience, I became less exuberant. "Let's talk when I get done with my shift," I said. "Where are you staying?"

"We're here as long as we keep selling sandals," he said, pointing to the van.

"OK, I'll be done in a few hours, and then we can go somewhere, get something to eat."

He nodded and gave me a thumbs-up. I hurried back into the emergency department. The nurses swarmed over me like angry wasps, stinging me with questions and problems as I walked from patient to patient. Who could be admitted? Why was the patient still here? Could they restrain the drunken man on the corner stretcher?

The drunken man snarled, spit, and pawed at me as I examined him. "Yes, restrain him," I said. "He's totally uncooperative. Why's he here?"

"Police brought him in. Found him drunk on the street. Store owners complained. He's too drunk for jail," Cindy said.

I looked for his chart. Alpha Doe was his name, because we had no real name for him. I wrote the restraint order and moved on to the other patients.

Ten minutes later I smelled smoke, and then the fire alarm went off. "It's Alpha Doe. He set himself on fire," said Cindy as she ran for a fire extinguisher.

"Evacuate the other patients!" I yelled as smoke filled the cubicles. I grabbed two interns. "Wheel those stretchers out to the waiting room," I said, pointing to two patients attached by wires to cardiac monitors, their anxious faces becoming obscured by the smoke.

I ran to see what was happening to Alpha Doe. Cindy was spraying him and his stretcher with fire-extinguisher foam. The smoke and foam filled the air, but I could see where Alpha Doe had burned himself on his ankle.

"He tried to burn off his restraints," she said. "Caught the mattress on fire." Then she held up a cigarette lighter. "He used this."

"All right, we'll have to treat his burns, but they don't look too bad," I said. "Let's get him out into the waiting room until the smoke clears out." So we put him on another stretcher and wheeled him out. I noticed that he was no longer spitting or fighting, as if his need for attention had been satisfied by this sudden flurry of activity.

"Jimmy," he said. "My name's Jimmy Duran."

"OK, Mr. Duran. You've got a burn on your ankle. We'll take care of it as soon as the smoke is gone."

Then the fire department arrived to check the mattress and look for any signs of fire or injuries. They dispersed through the emergency department with their axes and helmets and found one elderly lady who had been forgotten in a cubicle. When a fireman asked me about her, I said, "She's OK. She's just demented, and probably didn't realize what was going on. Can we bring the other patients back in?"

"Yeah, Doc, you're clear," said the fireman as he began to watch one of the televisions left on in a patient cubicle. "It's my favorite show."

When the patients were wheeled back to the cubicles, I looked more carefully at Alpha Doe—Jimmy Duran. He had a second-degree burn on his ankle, but remarkably little else.

"They tied me up. I was just trying to get out," he said as I examined his ankle. "Can I have a cigarette?"

"A cigarette?" I said. "Look what you've already done."

He shrugged.

My shift was over, and I explained to Mark, my replacement, why everything seemed so chaotic and confused. He nodded as if he had heard it all before.

When I got outside, a fire engine stood where Tony's van had been. The firemen were still checking to make sure the fire was contained. I looked around the hospital parking lot for Tony and his white van with California plates.

The lot was fairly packed with cars, considering it was a Saturday afternoon—pickups with gun racks, old dented Chevys with mismatched paint, lowriders with chrome wheels. I scanned the lot and walked to the far corner to get another perspective.

I felt him tap me on the shoulder before I saw him.

"Hey," I said, "I thought I lost you."

"The fire chief told us we were blocking a fire lane. There was a fire in the hospital, so we had to split."

"I know. The fire was in the emergency room. One of my patients set himself on fire."

"Oh man, that's like during the Vietnam War with those Buddhist priests. Burning while they just sat there."

"Well, it wasn't that bad. He burned only his foot, but we had to evacuate the emergency room."

"Man, that's wild," he said and patted me on the back.

"Where's your van? Let's go for a drink or something," I said.

"We're across the street at the sandwich shop," he said.

We crossed Lomas Boulevard, the six-lane street in front of the hospital, and sat down at a booth. With Tony out of the wind and sun, I could study his face. His brown eyes protruded from three layers of wrinkles, and a diamond stud earring glittered from his left earlobe. His shoulders and neck hung at an angle from his back, as if he had carried bags of cement on his shoulders for years, but his arms looked limber and muscular. After recovering from the initial shock of his appearance, I realized he had aged well. We ordered Cokes, and I asked him, "When did you start selling sandals?"

"Oh, it's just a little sideline. I go down to the clinic and pick up the sandals once or twice a year. I split the money with them. You know, they have this whole program now for disabled villagers."

"Yes, I read about it. But I didn't know you were still involved."

"Well, I've been back there off and on over the years, in between the mental hospital, jail, and a heart attack." He laughed.

"Really?" I asked.

"It's a long story," he said. "I found out I'm manic-depressive. They say the chemicals in my brain get messed up. Probably from all that acid I took. So I've got to take pills every day. I don't like them, but they keep me from getting too crazy."

"I never thought you were crazy," I said.

"Well, you didn't see me when I lived in the Black Mountain commune and worked on an organic farming movie for three weeks without sleeping or eating. Someone finally realized that I was messed up when I made salad out of my film."

"Oh, and whatever happened to your movie about the clinic? I saw a movie, but I didn't think it was yours," I said.

"Yeah, I spent months on that movie. But I just couldn't get it right. So I finally gave it to the foundation and told them to hire someone."

"So, are you making any movies?" I asked.

"Yeah, I got this gig going, a documentary about the farmworkers. I'll be filming next month."

"Great," I said. "And tell me about Kora."

"I'll let her mom tell you," he said, looking past me.

I turned my head and immediately noticed the legs, long and beautifully tapered. I followed them up to a face framed with long blond hair.

"Hi," she said, "I'm Jennifer."

"You remind me of someone," I said.

"That's what a lot of people say," she said. Her eyes became narrow slits as she smiled at me.

Tony took her hand and squeezed it. "Wasn't that what I told you when I met you?" he said, kissing Jennifer. "She's a healer-massager-acupressurist-channeler. You should let her work on you."

"Well, I could probably use it. Today was a bad day. A guy died, and I don't know but maybe we could have saved him. Then another patient set himself and the ER on fire. It was not one of my better days," I said.

"You need trauma reduction. There's a technique I'm learning that involves tapping on certain parts of the body, and it is unbelievable how well it removes stress or anxiety or guilt or trauma. There are connections between our nerves and brain that a few taps with your fingers will release," she said.

"Well, that sounds great," I said, trying to hide my skepticism. Her enthusiasm and earnestness kept me from refusing out of hand.

I had observed many unexplainable events in the emergency department over the years, but I had also resisted the new age alternative-healing procedures, like this tapping, that some of my patients described to me—usually as a treatment that they had tried before coming to the emergency department with appendicitis. They came too late, after the appendix had ruptured, and sometimes they almost died. But I was tired and frustrated and could feel my stomach churning as I thought about the day.

"OK," I said. "I could probably use it."

"Oh, yes, you definitely can," she said, and I could tell that she was delighted. "We need a quiet place. Let's go back to the van. We'll be done in a few minutes."

I looked at Tony, who nodded at me and gave a thumbs-up.

"I'll be right back," I said as we headed out of the restaurant to the van.

The inside of the van was like a disordered nest, with clothes and sandals piled onto a mattress with blankets. Jennifer quickly cleared a spot for us to sit, and she began to explain the technique.

"You tap three times above your right eyebrow, then on your chest below the clavicle, then tap on your little finger. That's to deal with trauma, anxiety, and guilt."

"OK," I said.

"But first visualize something that makes you anxious, some trauma."

"OK," I said.

"What is it?" she asked.

"Well, I'm thinking about this guy today, hit by a car. He's gasping for air and asks me if he's going to die. And I tell him that he'll be okay now. We'll take care of him, not to worry. And he relaxes a bit and thanks me. But then we try to intubate him, and he dies. And I see his face staring up at me as I call the code. And in his face is reflected all the other faces over the years—the people who died or suffered in front of me. And then I see them decomposing into a gray shimmering column of smoke that fills the ER, and I'm coughing and choking, and I run from the smoke until I realize it's coming from my patient Alpha Doe—Jimmy Duran—so I run back and pull him out while he spits on me, and then I collapse."

"Anything else?"

"Well, things are not great at home," I said. I blurted it out without thinking, because that's what I had been feeling lately, when I came home.

"What do you mean?"

"I don't know. Sometimes my wife will say things—strange, hurtful things—and I don't know why. She says she needs space, her own space; that she is suffocating. And I get scared that I'm going to lose her and don't know what to do. And it's like the smoke in the emergency room. I'm afraid, but I have to go back in and rescue the children and her too."

"OK. Well, I'm not sure we can do all of that in one session, but we can try," she said.

"Now tap over your right eyebrow. You better do it five times. There's a lot of trauma," she said.

So I tapped with my index finger. Each tap sounded like a gavel in my ears, as if a judge were bringing order to a noisy, chaotic courtroom.

"Now tap five times just below your clavicle, just above your heart. Five times again," she said.

As I tapped, I waited for something to happen—some feeling or some sense of a weight being lifted from me. I looked at Jennifer and could see the intensity of her concentration, in her taut cheek and jaw muscles and pushed-out lips. She was breathing deeply and exhaling with an audible sigh.

"OK. Now tap five times on the medial side of the little finger of your left hand."

After I finished I waited for more instructions, but Jennifer now grinned at me. Her concentration had relaxed. "Well, you did it," she said. "How do you feel?"

"I don't know. About the same."

She frowned. "Do you still feel the anxiety? The guilt?"

"I'm still afraid that Laura, my wife, will leave me. She wants me to let go, but I can't."

"You must let go," she said, and I closed my eyes and breathed deeply. "Good," she said. "We need to amplify and consolidate." And she repeated her instructions about tapping above the eyebrow, heart, and finger.

As I repeated the sequence, I thought about how we marked the passage of time with clocks and rhythmic counting like this tapping. With each tap, I recalled a past event, a person, a time. I remembered the village, the woman with tetanus, the children with whooping cough, the músico—and all the others bleeding from the head or with bullet wounds in the chest, gasping for air, dying in front of me. I saw the matrimonial bed empty. And I saw my family, my colleagues, the nurses, the dean, and the hospital board all swirling past.

"How do you feel?" Jennifer asked.

"Better," I lied.

"Good," she said. "This works all the time."

We left the van and walked back into the restaurant to join Tony. Jennifer told me about her life; Kora, her daughter; and her quest to find a balance in her life.

Tony said it was time to go. The vibes weren't right anymore—the fire engines that forced them to move had been a message.

"Could you lend us some money?" he asked. "I'll send it back to you. We're a little short."

"Sure. How much do you need?"

"Whatever you can spare. Fifty, a hundred."

I looked in my wallet and pulled out three twenties.

"Thanks, man," he said. "I love you."

They piled into the van, and then they were gone.

As I walked to my car, I passed a man with crutches, hopping along the sidewalk. It was Alpha Doe—Jimmy Duran—his burned foot bandaged in gauze. We nodded in acknowledgment that we had met before.

"Spare a quarter?" he asked.

I reached into my pocket, but it was empty.

"Sorry," I said.

"No problem," he said.

Chapter Twenty-six

THE MEMORY OF TONY'S VISIT MADE ME SMILE. HE HAD survived crises, failures, disasters of all kinds, and here he was —traveling, enjoying the world, selling sandals. He had lived a disorganized, unfocused life, so different from mine; he had broken every rule that I thought essential, and now here we were, with his life happier than mine. Apparently Carl's influence on him had not caused any harm. We didn't even talk about Carl. We never brought up that time in the darkroom. With each passing year, I began to think that maybe Carl would get away with it, and that maybe he had stopped. Sometimes as people get older, sexual feelings evolve into religious or spiritual feelings, and they stop expressing them physically. And so, a few years later when I was in the desert in Utah and finally heard about the allegations, I expected them and yet was surprised.

Because of my administrative role as chairman of emergency medicine, I would often receive requests to serve as a consultant in other states. I never made a conscious decision to become a chairman, and my transformation had happened gradually as I spent more time in meetings and less time in the emergency department with patients. It was as if a new thick film was growing over my skin, insulating me from the raw emotional reactions of sick patients and changing my language and thought processes. Perhaps one of the compensations for the boring and frustrating meetings I had to attend was the opportunity to consult. Usually I'd decline, because I worried about leaving home, as if something might happen. But when the offer to visit a nerve-gas storage facility arrived, I agreed to go. I was curious about the place and the people who worked there.

The storage facility was in a valley that lay hidden between mountains and the Great Salt Lake. It was only an hour from Salt Lake City, and yet it felt rural and untouched, serene—at least until the barbed wire fence and warning signs announced the presence of something else hidden down in the valley. I had come to this place willingly as a consultant on emergency medicine preparedness, drawn by a fascination with the secrets that had flourished here for years.

We all think about dying sometimes. And I thought about dying when I saw the cement bunkers that stored the "agent." They never called it poison or nerve gas or sarin, just "agent." I imagined what the symptoms would be: sweating and the overload of nervous impulses leading to collapse. Perhaps it was the heat, but I noticed that I was already perspiring down my forehead and under my arms.

We stopped at a wooden building for our mask fittings. Two of the men had beards and had to shave them. Inside the building was an airtight chamber. When I entered the chamber, I saw a sheet of paper with paragraphs in English and Russian, which were meant to be read during the fitting process as a banana-scented gas mixture was pumped into the chamber. "Do you smell anything?" asked the technician.

"No." I shook my head, because the mask was working, keeping the gas from entering my nose or mouth.

Then the technician asked me to read the statement in English. I read it and realized that breathing in the mask was restricted, even uncomfortable. The mask provided necessary, if incomplete, protection.

"Why the Russian?" I asked after my fitting.

"Russia and the United States have to monitor each other's supplies of nerve gas," said Tom, our earnest, balding guide. "When we fit the Russians with a mask, they read the Russian."

"Oh, vestiges of the cold war." I smiled.

My guide nodded without smiling. "And here's an atropine injector kit," he said as he demonstrated how you could jab it into your thigh in seconds, before you lost consciousness.

"Great," I said.

We entered a room where various samples of missiles, land mines, and shells were displayed. Tom picked up a small shell.

"Should we put on our masks?" I asked.

"No, this is just a display model. It does not contain agent." He clutched the shell to his chest lovingly, as one might hold a young child. Then he passed it around quickly.

Gary, one of my fellow consultants, came up to me. We had worked together in Costa Rica years before, to assess the country's EMS (emergency medical services) system. Now, without his beard, he looked vulnerable and anxious.

"My wife has never seen me without a beard," he said.

"Quite a sacrifice," I said.

"Yeah, but I had to see it. Can you believe these guys? They're fossils from the fifties," he said, pointing to our guide. "This might as well be another country."

Then, as we began to descend into the tunnel that led to the incinerator, he said, "Didn't you once work at that clinic in Mexico with Carl Wilson?"

"Yes," I said, knowing that the clinic was so famous now for its innovative approach to community development, that I would not need to say anything more to describe it.

We passed an air lock and a warning sign about testing our masks.

"I just read about it in the newspaper," he said. "I'm sure you've heard about it."

"What?" I asked, as I tried to slow my breathing.

"Well, the paper said that Carl Wilson had been abusing Mexican boys for twenty years. Having sex with them. He's been fired from the clinic."

"Oh. Well, I hadn't heard about it, but I guess I'm not that surprised," I said, shaken, breathing too fast. "It was a long time ago. And there was this boy, Luis. But I don't know if it was really abuse," I said.

"What do you mean?" he asked.

I could hardly concentrate as I passed through shiny metallic cylinders, clutching my antidotes. "It was sort of an . . . arrangement they had. It didn't seem so bad. And you know Carl was doing such great stuff, saving people's lives, bringing medicine and supplies to the people, bringing kids to the United States for treatment and education. I mean, he was like a god down there." I was gasping as I finished, the words rushing out. And I became more anxious as I realized I was defending Carl without even knowing what he had done.

"The paper said a volunteer claimed that Carl Wilson had molested more than twenty boys, some as young as eleven years old. Someone from the foundation called the newspapers."

"Really?" I pounded the antidote syringe against the wall and liquid antidote came spraying out as if to counteract the poisonous conversation around me. Gary watched for a moment as I dropped the used syringe into a wastebasket.

"But none of the boys will come forward and give evidence. And Wilson denies it. Says he was just helping them, like a mentor," he said.

I nodded and bent down to tie my shoe. Gary moved on ahead of me, and our conversation ended. I was thinking about all the years that we volunteers all knew and wondering why the allegations had become public now, and whether one of the boys would come forward and describe what had happened. And what if no one did? What was my responsibility? It had been so long ago, and I really didn't know much. What I did know worried me—that maybe it was true that he was still abusing boys—and I felt touched by it, complicit. I felt like it contaminated everything else we had done, all the lives we'd saved.

We headed into the incinerator. The tubes of metal through which the gases would flow curved and turned at riveted connecting joints. I followed the path of nerve gas flushing through a giant plumbing system. A computerized tracking system that was manned twenty-four hours a day monitored temperature, air quality, and every movement of anything living or mechanical in the tunnels. Warning signs at every door reminded me of the lethal contents. A siren and loudspeaker could be instantly activated by the computer system. Tom, our guide, supplied details about temperatures, scrubbers, alarms, and gas monitors. At the end of our tour, as I was returning my mask, he took me aside.

"Well, what do you think you guys are going to say?"

"I don't know. It's impressive, but I'm not sure about the safety."

"Yeah, now that we built this incinerator, I guess we have to use it unless you fellas say we can't." He winked.

"Well, it's pretty dangerous stuff to be stored around here. There's really no need for it, now that the Russians are destroying their supplies."

"Yeah, I guess not," Tom said. "Just the same, I'm glad we've had it here all these years. Sort of like a gun under your pillow; helps you get to sleep." He smiled.

I walked out into the searing desert sun to a car that would take me away. Large black flies buzzed around my head, and I remembered that the nerve gas had been invented to eliminate them and other insects.

Tom waved to me as our car passed the security checkpoint, and I could imagine him sleeping soundly, a loaded gun tucked under his pillow. And then my mind drifted back to Carl, his secret exposed. I raised my hand to swat at a black fly that had gotten into our car and was frantically darting against the window. Then I opened the window and watched as it disappeared toward the bunkers of nerve gas.

Chapter Twenty-seven

AS I WAS ABOUT TO LEAVE THE OFFICE, THERE WAS A KNOCK at the door. It was Rick.

"You still here?" he asked.

"Yeah, I was sort of daydreaming," I said.

"I just remembered something about that place in Mexico. I read it in the papers," he said.

"What's that?" I asked.

"That place you want to go to in Mexico—isn't that the place I read about? The guy was a pervert. He was doing it with young boys. Wasn't that the place?" Rick asked.

"Yeah," I said, "there was an article about it in the paper. It was never proven."

"But you must have known if it was going on. People don't make that kind of stuff up."

"Well, you know, it was the sixties or the early seventies, and Americans would come down to the village to volunteer, and sometimes there would be these little relationships. Mostly, it was the Mexican guys and the American girls. Occasionally, one of the American guys would have a village girlfriend. But this guy, Carl, who was in charge of the clinic, was pretty discrete. He had this one Mexican boy, a teenager, who I guess had a relationship with him. Mostly they were companions, and everyone seemed to accept it. I was maybe twenty or twenty-two at the time. You know how you are at that age, your mind jumping around reading sexual intentions into actions that don't have them, getting turned on at inopportune moments, analyzing your sexual thoughts, worrying about them. I just figured I was being uptight even wondering about it."

"Did he come on to you?"

"To me? No, I was too old."

"Too old. You were what, in your twenties? How old was he?"

"I don't know, maybe thirty-five or forty."

"And you were too old?"

"Yeah, I heard he liked them younger, thirteen or fourteen."

"That's sick. That guy should be in jail. Are you going to see him when you go down there?"

"I don't think so. He doesn't go there very much anymore. I'm mostly going to see the other people—the family I lived with and some of the others from the village. And I want to see what the place looks like."

"How did he keep from getting caught?"

"I don't know," I said.

"I'm not proud of everything I did," said Rick. "There were times I got drunk and ended up in bed with someone, and I had no memory of it. Sometimes you mess up. Particularly when you're a young buck. But there has to be a line somewhere. I'd kill anyone who touched my kids. Doesn't matter if I ended up in jail. I'd get a gun and kill the motherfucker myself."

"Yeah, I know what you mean. I feel the same way about my kids. But this guy really seemed to be in another world, making new rules. The whole mood of the place was to question what was going on in the old world and do things differently."

"Yeah, it sounds like he was doing things differently. Sounds like some kind of sexual Disneyland with a different ride for every taste."

"No, Rick, it wasn't like that. Mostly everyone just worked in the clinic and took care of sick people. If you live somewhere day after day, night after night, you become friends, and in some cases it gets deeper. It wasn't only in one direction. I think people realized there were advantages in marrying an American and getting out of the village to the United States."

"So what's the appeal of going back? Sounds like everyone wants to get out. They'll even sleep with you to do it."

"No, not everyone. But for some people, our life here looks so exciting with so much possibility. And life there was pretty hard and pretty predictable."

"I wonder what that guy is doing now. Maybe he's down there hiding out, and you'll find him."

"I doubt it. But who knows, I might bump into him."

"He'll probably be some pathetic old senile guy. He probably won't even remember any of it."

"Yeah," I said, "like Reagan, who said he couldn't remember that he had authorized all those guys to break the law, and then he really was senile. There are certain memories that are too dangerous or painful to remember. They pull at you like a flame, but then if you get too close, it hurts."

"Well, be careful down there. We don't want you getting sick and missing shifts when you get back," said Rick, and he opened the door to leave my office.

As he was exiting, I heard him greet someone at the door. "Dave, you have a visitor," he said.

A woman poked her head into the office. She had long auburn hair and dark eyes and was wearing a gray and white dress. "Hi," she said. "I had these brownies for my staff nurses upstairs, and they told me to get rid of them because they are all on diets."

Rick interrupted her. "Dave, do you know Peggy Norman? She's one of the internal medicine clinic doctors. She is also a dancing instructor." Rick laughed.

"Oh, yes, I do know Peggy," I said. "She sent me the nicest e-mail a few days ago."

Peggy smiled and said, "I hope I can leave you these brownies."

"Sure, sure. In emergency medicine we're always snacking. The residents will gobble them up in minutes."

"Well, I'll leave you two," said Rick, winking at me.

"Uh, come in," I said to Peggy.

She sat down, the brownies in her lap.

"I can only stay for a minute. We have patients upstairs."

"Yeah, I've got all of these evaluations to do," I said, pointing to the stack of papers on my desk. We looked at each other for a moment, and I tried to remember if I had seen her before. She looked familiar, but also different. Perhaps it was her hair. "Thanks for that e-mail," I said. "It came at a moment when I needed a lift."

"Well, we don't give much positive feedback here," she said. "I wanted you to know how much I respected what you did."

"How do you like being on the executive committee?" I asked.

"Oh, well, for me it's an eye-opener. I'm only an at-large member, so no one expects me to know anything, but I am amazed at how all those intelligent people can sit there month after month and do so little. But the lunches are good." She smiled.

"Well, thanks for the brownies. I'll treat you to a two-for-one café mocha at the coffee cart," I said.

"I'd like that."

"Good. Then it's a deal. I'll call you."

She left the brownies on the chair and walked out the door.

I looked at the brownies sitting on the chair. I picked them up and carried them out to the hallway for the residents and visitors.

Chapter Twenty-eight

AFTER PEGGY NORMAN LEFT, I FINISHED LOOKING AT MY mail, signed a few memos, and decided to go home. After I parked in my driveway and went into the house, I decided to go for a jog along the dirt trails near the river. Large cottonwood trees created shade from the summer heat, and I looked forward to the exercise and change of my thoughts. When I ran out in the woods, I had to concentrate on the uneven ground, the roots extending across the trail, little ruts, and small rocks. My mind had to release all the problems of the day.

As I turned the corner from my driveway and headed to the woods, one of the neighbors waved to me. He was cutting down weeds and trimming back bushes.

I waved back, and he motioned me to come over.

"Hi, Joe," I said.

"Hi," he said. "I want to let you know that I was the one who sent the newsman over to your house. He had been asking me about the house for years. He almost bought it at the time that you and your wife got it, and I think he never forgot about it. So when I heard your wife moved out, I thought you might be needing to sell. Sorry if I was mixing into your personal business. He's an old friend of mine. He comes on a bit strong, but he's a good guy."

"Well, I was surprised. But I guess I do need to think about it. And maybe I will sell it; I don't know. Everything is a bit jumbled for me," I said.

"I understand," he said. "I've been divorced. She left me after twenty years. Told me she didn't want to be married anymore. It was the strangest thing. I never saw it coming. But she had it all planned out and wanted me to move out to a hotel that night."

"So did you move out?" I asked.

"No. I told her that we had company coming over, and she got all flustered and started cooking, and we didn't even talk about it again for a week. Then she moved out and left me a note about feeding the dog and watering the plants and didn't tell me where she was going."

"Wow, that's strange," I said.

"Would you like to come in for a drink?" he asked.

"Well, I'm heading out for a run," I said. "Maybe another time."

When I got back to the house, I found a letter and a note on the kitchen table from Laura. I hadn't noticed them earlier when I came home. "David, I hope you're holding up. I wanted you to know my new phone number." And the note outlined all of the pertinent information—the number and her address. Then I opened the letter.

I know this is hard for you, for both of us, but I trust that we will come out of this the better for the experience. I believe that things happen for a reason. Our relationship is just evolving into a new phase, an independent phase, and we will both be able to grow in ways that we could not when we were together. Please call next time before you visit my new place. I have rooms for the children, and I'm sure they will be comfortable in both homes.

Fondly,
Laura

I folded the letter and put it into my pocket. I thought about the story my neighbor had told me and the sudden unfolding of events now in my life. For so many years, everything had gone along fairly predictably, and our lives had attained a rhythm that felt comfortable. I had thought we were happy and not too different from most other families. Mexico and the people I had known there reappeared only in my bedtime stories to my children or in my dreams. But I did not know much about Laura's dreams. Perhaps they had begun to exist during the daylight hours.

Over the next two weeks, I showed up for my emergency department shifts on time, attended meetings, shopped for groceries, paid the bills, and waited for a response to my letter to Rosa and Ricardo. I had addressed it to them, using their names and the village and state, but no street name. The street still had not been named, and the people at the post office knew where Ricardo and Rosa lived. Letters to people arrived at the post office, which was located in another village an hour away. They would accumulate there until someone from the village would deliver the mail by hand. Sometimes a letter would sit for days, and sometimes it was opened by a curious neighbor or postal worker looking for money. Until I got a letter back, I could not go, and the time I had planned for the trip was almost here. Finally, after two weeks, a letter arrived from Mexico.

David,

How happy we feel to receive your letter. We always think of you and what happened to you. We are waiting for your arrival with great joy. We are all well. The clinic is very pretty, and you will like everything and have a wonderful time here. Our children are all married except the youngest, who received her engineering degree three months ago. Work is hard, and there is much to talk about. Make sure and practice your Spanish. For all my children I want to say come. Only Victor, our youngest son, lives with us now. Otherwise we are alone. Come for several days to improve your Spanish. We hope you understand our letter.

Greetings and we await you.
Rosa and Ricardo

The plane trip through Phoenix felt strange. Everyone was dressed in either suits or beach clothes, and I wondered if I had made a mistake in going. I still was not sure what I expected to find or how I would know if I found it.

I landed in Mazatlán and rented a car. It was early June, when the heat was oppressive and before the rains began. Driving along the two-lane road that led to the village, I concentrated on each hairpin turn. I patiently passed slow-moving trucks and buses, but once I spotted signs to the village, I felt my heart quicken.

Men on muleback in long-sleeved shirts and broad-brimmed hats waved as I passed. I was surprised to see younger men, teenagers, and young boys wearing baseball caps—some turned backward in the style commonly worn in the United States. As the road turned to dirt, the boulders jutting up from low spots scraped the underside of the car, and I slowed down.

The road made a dip and then rose past the first houses of the village. A man walking up the road and carrying a machete stared into the car, and our eyes locked for a brief moment of recognition. I nodded, desperately trying to match his face with my memories. Finally I remembered that I had treated him for tuberculosis over many months when I was at the clinic. He used to come every week for injections of streptomycin, often carrying his machete. We would disappear behind a white sheet hanging from a rope, where he would lower his trousers, and I would select an area of his smooth brown buttocks for the needle. He never flinched or complained, and he thanked me as he returned to his field. I was long past him before I remembered that he had a parrot that used to say his name, "Berto, Berto."

The road curved past a group of small houses thick with the smoke of the evening meal, to a square where several men and teenage boys stood in groups talking and joking. They turned to stare at me as I drove by. I recognized Ricardo and Rosa's house on the next corner and parked in front. Before I could get out of the car, Rosa appeared at my window, a broad smile exposing her gold front teeth. She peered in at me with delight and amazement, as if the winds had deposited a treasure on her doorstep.

I got out and we hugged. Rosa had become thinner and looked frail. She shuffled as she walked, but her dimples and bright eyes glowed. She said "Qué David" over and over as she had when I lived in her house, and she wiped at her dark eyes with a crumpled tissue. Ricardo arrived and shook my hand. He had gained a lot of weight, which he carried mostly in his stomach, but his shoulders and arms still looked powerful. They were arms made to grip a rope and not let go. Or perhaps it was the man connected to the arms. His eyes had lost some of their brightness, and they even suggested a tinge of sadness. We stood in the road outside the house looking at each other, a small crowd gathering around us. He rocked on his bootheels and shook his head as he stared at me.

"Your wife?" he asked.

"Not here," I said. He nodded and did not pursue the question further.

Thunder rumbled through the valley, shaking the adobe walls and stopping our conversation. We moved to an area under the overhanging roof outside the door to their house. It was a sort of porch with five chairs standing against the wall that faced the street. We used to sit there with men from the upper villages before dinner, sipping on sodas. The chairs now were white plastic, like lawn furniture, except for one rough-hewn wooden survivor of the past. I remembered the chairs in a semicircle, Ricardo in the middle, a few words of conversation, great gaps of silence, and another sprinkle of words. The conversations were like the geography: long trails without people, then a cluster of five or six houses, then another long empty trail and a few more houses.

A blinding flash of light preceded the initial drops of rain.

"The first rain," said Ricardo as we watched the large drops kick up the dust in the road. "We need this rain. You've brought us good luck." The storm passed after a half hour of hard rain, and the air felt fresh and clean. "Pase," Ricardo said, leading me into the house for dinner.

A table set for three waited under a naked light bulb that glowed from the wall. Rosa and Ricardo and I ate the beans with hot fresh corn tortillas from the stove and wiped our plates clean. When we finished, another set of diners appeared to replace us—a son, now in his thirties, who helped Ricardo with the ranching; his two young children and wife; another young woman, whose family lived in the mountains, and who stayed with Ricardo and Rosa while attending school; and then several other villagers who seemed to appear at the right time and were invited to eat. I remembered the custom that if someone appeared at dinnertime, you were obligated to offer them food. It was an informal system for the poor, in which Ricardo and Rosa participated proudly.

After dinner Ricardo and I sat quietly in front of the house. Except for an occasional lumbering truck, the street was quiet.

"Ricardo," I asked, "do you mind if I ask you about some old friends?"

"Certainly, if I know them."

"What about Demetrio and his family—do you remember them? I visited them once in their village, in Chilar."

Ricardo shifted in his chair and folded his arms. His words came slowly and quietly. "Something very bad happened in their village. There are no people living in that place anymore."

"What happened? Are they dead?"

"Dead."

"All of them."

"Yes, all of them." His voice trailed off. We sat in silence while I thought about what to say next. He didn't seem to want to tell me more. His face had tightened and solidified as he looked down at his hands and stretched his thick fingers.

"And your children?"

"All fine," he said, relaxing gradually. He told me that Tomás, the oldest, lived in a neighboring village. He suggested that maybe I could see him the next day, when he had to transport pigs to that village for sale.

"Very well," I said. I had always expected Tomás would take over Ricardo's ranching operation. He loved to be out on horseback in the mountains. I was surprised to hear that he lived in a neighboring village rather than in Ricardo's house.

We talked of other changes in the village. The electricity that powered the lights, the water that flowed from a spigot every morning, the airplane that flew people to the upper villages in fifteen minutes rather than the twelve hours required for ground travel. But the plane flew out of another village, and the traffic that used to pass through now went to the other village. He showed me his television, a small box that remained on constantly.

"Very pretty," I said, trying to hide my disappointment that television had come to the village. I realized that I had hoped to escape from the tumultuous changes in my own life to a place with familiar sights and sounds that had resisted change. I yearned for the storytelling and singing that used to follow dinner. But talk could not compete with the flashy television images. His grandchildren stared silently at the glittering box. Finally I decided to ask about Carl. "How about don Carlos? Have you seen him recently?"

"Yes, he was here last month. You just missed him. He seems to be well."

I felt both disappointment and relief. I had no idea what I would say to him, but I wanted to see him anyway.

As I sat with Ricardo, it became late, and my eyes began to close.

"The bed has been prepared," he said, and he led me into the room with a bed, a fan, and a crucifix on the wall. He and Rosa had slept in this room for more than forty years. They had insisted that Laura and I sleep there when we had visited years before. And he had no hesitation in donating it to me for this night. No arguments from me could dissuade him. Ricardo and Rosa would sleep in cots in the hallway.

As I tried to sleep, the memories of my last time in that bed swirled in my head, and the unfamiliar sounds of the house kept waking me up. When I woke up in the night, I remembered lying there years before with Laura, our life extending out before us with possibilities. I tried to stretch my legs out to find her. It seemed that she had been there with me only a moment before. But I couldn't reach her; she was too far away. The bed was too big for me. As I tried to find a comfortable spot, I turned and tossed, the sheets got twisted around my neck, and I woke with a start as the roosters began to crow.

The next morning we had breakfast. Tortillas with beans and rice. I ate hungrily, enjoying the familiarity of the kitchen and the food. Not much had changed over the years. Electricity, running water, but the food tasted the same. After gobbling down the tortillas, I decided to take a quick walk around the village.

"I'll be back in a little while," I said, and Ricardo and Rosa nodded without questioning me.

I walked down the street past Luis's house. It was quiet now. I used to wave to his parents, but no one was sitting outside the door now. I wondered how Luis had been the chosen one. Was it his enthusiasm, good looks, willingness to serve, courage, optimism? The lives of most people remained on the prescribed trail with uncertainties about the time and nature of marriage, birth, and death but otherwise bounded by the realities of life in the village. But not Luis. He had escaped into another world, and Carl had been the vital link that had made it possible. Paint was peeling off the façade of Luis's house, and the door remained closed as if no one was yet awake. I continued along the main street of the village. I waved at people who were staring suspiciously at me. A few waved back hesitantly. I had walked this street before and wondered how many of the same people had been here then: perhaps the old man stooped over with arthritis, perhaps the fat woman hurrying home with an armful of vegetables. Perhaps some of them had been my patients. But my life had diverged from their lives long ago. And this brief visit was as inconsequential to them as the lighting of a fly upon a window.

A man carrying two bales of straw appeared on the road in front of me. All I could see were legs and feet; his head and torso had been replaced by straw. No head, no stomach, just feet striding ahead. Sometimes I felt like that, like my body had been cut away and replaced with a heavy, ungainly load that threatened to come apart or topple me as I carried it. My home, my job, my family, all fastened to my legs, and I wondered if anyone could see me underneath it all. I carried it because I had to. And I felt a sense of accomplishment when I finally arrived. I was relieved not to have dropped anyone. But was that enough, to arrive at my destination in spite of the obstacles and the load? What about the destination itself? As I watched the feet with straw disappear into a store, a toddler stumbled out of a doorway in front of me and began to cry. When I bent to pick him up, a man with wild eyes and a thick moustache scooped him away and clutched the baby to his chest.

We stared at each other, and I knew the man did not trust me; perhaps he even imagined I might do something to harm his baby. I wanted to tell him his baby was safe with me, that I was a doctor. But I knew it was useless, and I turned and walked away.

I passed the house of doña Mercedes. She had often sat just outside the door, waving her frail hand when I passed by on my way to visit a patient. I remembered how her high-pitched cackle and yelled suggestions had unnerved me when I tried to pull teeth. Her house now seemed pale and lifeless.

Finally, I turned up an alley and returned to Ricardo's house.

Ricardo was waiting there.

"I have to sell two pigs," said Ricardo. "If you would like to see Tomás, I can take you with the pigs in the truck now."

I wanted to see Tomás, Ricardo's oldest son. He had been eleven when I first arrived in the village, and he always loved to work with his father in the field.

The pigs squealed and struggled as we lifted them into the truck. We had buckets of water to keep them cool in the heat. But they still suffered from the bouncing and the unfamiliar truck bottom, and their squeals upset me. Ricardo drove us to a small, pink house on a narrow street. Tomás was standing outside with a small child. He wore jeans and a straw hat. He had the beginnings of a middle-aged paunch and the same powerful shoulders as his father.

"Hola, David," he said as I jumped out of the truck, and he squeezed me in a bear hug.

"Hi, Tomás." We stood together for a moment, and then Ricardo excused himself, saying he'd be back in an hour.

"Pase, David," Tomás said, directing us into his house. A pungent-smelling candle burned in the foyer, and the house had a somber feel.

"Oh, David," he said, "it's been so hard."

"What has?" I asked.

"Didn't my father tell you about the kidnapping?" he asked.

"No," I said. "He told me everything was fine."

"Well, he doesn't like to think about it. But men with guns kidnapped me in the mountains near El Chilar. I was checking on some cattle." He paused. "There were six men, and they tied me to a tree and kicked me and held a gun to my ear. They wanted half a million pesos, about sixty thousand American dollars, from my parents. Imagine, sixty thousand dollars! Even if we sold everything we owned, we could not reach sixty thousand dollars."

"Oh, Tomás, why didn't your parents tell me?"

"Probably they didn't want you to pity them or become scared."

"So then what happened?"

"My parents sold everything. All of my relatives got loans and sold what they could, and finally they paid the money."

"Did you know who the kidnappers were?" I asked.

"Yes," he said, "I knew them. Their bodies smell like a rotten goat. They smoke marijuana and have yellow teeth. They are cowards, except when they are together. But they are also crazy. And because I know them—that's what keeps me awake at night. Because I can still feel the gun in my ear and feel the punches and the kicks."

As I listened to Tomás repeat parts of his story, his wife brought small, brown fruits for us to eat. "The violence is horrible," he said. "You cannot go into the mountains without your own army. Someone will kidnap you, take the ransom money, and still kill you. There have been other kidnappings. Two boys from the village were killed even though their parents paid money. Nobody is safe anymore." He spoke calmly, dripping fruit juice from his lips.

"Is that what happened to Demetrio's family?"

"We don't know, David," he said. "We don't know what happened. They were our friends. Demetrio, his brother, the children, and the wives. And still no one knows what happened. They are gone. We think they are dead, buried somewhere in the mountains. They just disappeared one day. The house is empty. Every day is a nightmare for me. Nothing is safe anymore. Even in the brightness of the day I am afraid."

And then Tomás stood up and cried. I stood up and hugged him again and imagined the pain he must be feeling to act like this in front of me. I cried too, for him and for myself and for everything that had happened to us. Then I shook his hand. At least he was not dead, like Demetrio. It was a shocking story, and I could only shake my head in disbelief. When Ricardo came, we stopped crying and tried to smile.

I left with Ricardo, and we drove back to the village in silence. As we passed the clinic, I said, "I'd like to visit the clinic." Tomás's story had pried the lid off my images from the past, and I needed to see what existed now.

"The clinic is finished," he said. "Gabriel has a small pharmacy, but the clinic is finished." He said this without bitterness, and I remembered his letter, which had painted a very different picture. Why had he misled me?

I walked over to the building. The sign for the clinic had disappeared and in its place a new sign proclaimed *Farmacia.* Gabriel looked up at me from behind a counter and hurried to his feet. He sported a great black beard. "David, how great to see you," he said. He squeezed my hand, and I could feel the rheumatoid joints sticking as they attempted to move.

I remembered teaching Gabriel about the books and medicines years ago as he taught me Spanish. Carl had not initially recognized his potential and his motivation. But I knew that with his severe rheumatoid arthritis, Gabriel would not be able to do other physically demanding labor. And so I gave him a chance. Now here he was, the last vestige of the project.

"So you are the clinic now," I said.

"Well, the clinic is actually finished. I run a small pharmacy here, but we don't have any doctors for the clinic," he said. "But the government has a clinic and a doctor. People go there now."

"Could I walk through the building?" I asked.

"Sure, let me get the key."

The rooms were filthy, covered with bird droppings, dirt, and feathers. The books that were piled in corners were mildewed and stained. A suitcase lay open in the loft, its contents of clothes spilled out. As I moved from room to room, I felt like I was examining the decaying body of an old friend. Finally, I saw the old picture that Carl had drawn—the two hands floating in space, now covered with dirt and discarded in a pile.

"I remember when we used to get visitors from all over the United States," I said.

"People still come from all over the world," he said. "India, Japan, and the Philippines."

I didn't know what to say, because I realized there was nothing for a visitor to see now. It would be a wasted trip. The dream of the clinic and all the books and articles were frozen in the past with the old clothes and rotting papers. Gabriel and I returned to the pharmacy, where a tall, slim man with clanging silver spurs conferred with Gabriel about a cough. I watched as Gabriel examined the man, listened with his stethoscope, and handed the man white pills wrapped in paper. The man paid Gabriel twenty pesos, and Gabriel bought us Cokes with the money. We sipped them slowly. "What heat," I said. "I can't stop sweating."

"Maybe you are being too active," he said.

"Yes, well, I only have a few days here, and I wanted to see everyone, maybe take a horseback ride along the river. So how about you? Will you continue as a pharmacist?"

"I don't know. The clinic has closed, and I don't know if there will be enough money to support my family and me. And the violence has been getting worse. Last month three men were shot in the village. And perhaps you know about Tomás's kidnapping."

"Yes."

"But Carlos is thinking of starting a new project against violence. He says it's worse than all the diarrhea and pneumonia we used to have. People are leaving the village because they don't feel safe. And I worry about my children too."

Gabriel asked me about my work at the university. I told him that I taught emergency medicine.

"You were my first teacher," he said.

"And you were my first student," I said. His eyes lit up.

Then I changed the subject to Carl, who had taught us both. I wondered how much Gabriel knew about the alleged abuse, and how he felt about it.

"Gabriel, you know that Carl has been cut off from the foundation that supported the clinic," I said. "There were allegations that he had sexual relations with boys from the village."

"Yes, I know about that. Several Americans came here and asked questions, but nobody would talk to them." He smiled with satisfaction as he explained this to me.

"People are very loyal to Carl," I said.

"Como no. He has helped every family in the village at one time or another. And he has been coming here for many years." He reviewed some of Carl's accomplishments: the clinic; a grain bank; a drinking-water system; education of village children in medicine, dentistry, agriculture, and pharmacy; the rehabilitation program for spinal cord injuries; and travel to all parts of the world for villagers who helped Carl.

It was an impressive list that contrasted sharply with the current neglected state of the clinic and the projects. But like the intelligence and compassion hidden inside Gabriel's arthritic body, the clinic continued to emit a glow of idealism and hope from all the good that had been accomplished, even as the walls deteriorated. I finished my Coke, thanked Gabriel, and walked back to Ricardo's house. He was sitting quietly facing the street, and I found a place next to him.

"Ricardo," I said, "I heard about Tomás."

"I didn't want to bother you with this and frighten you," he said, pausing to look up at the sky. "We had to sell everything, and even then it was not enough." He paused again. "So Rosa wrote to don Carlos, and he got the money and drove for two days and brought it to us. Then Rosa had a dream that Tomás was dead. I prayed to God all night, and finally just before dawn a voice told me that Tomás was alive, but we would have to give up everything for him to be returned to us. And I said I would give up everything, even my life. Because they are only things. So I am not sad. I am happy. I have seen the love of my children and friends and I have my son. And with God's help, we will rebuild our life better than it was before."

"I didn't know that Carl had brought the money for you," I said.

"Yes, he is part of my family—like you, David," and he leaned over and hugged me. "And David, what about you?"

"Oh, Ricardo, it's been difficult. My wife moved out of my house."

"Here," he said, "a wife would not leave her husband's house unless he beat her."

"No, I would never do that," I said. "In the United States it's different. People leave when they're not happy. She wanted a new life. I was afraid to lose the life that I had, and she was afraid of losing herself. Sometimes we don't know what's most important in our lives. But you knew that. You gave everything you owned for Tomás, but you will rebuild your life. I don't know how I will rebuild mine. I don't even know where to begin."

He nodded. "We're all family. All of the people who have lived in my house, all of my children and their children, all of the people who are in my heart and Rosa's heart—we are all family." He paused to think for a moment. "David," he continued, "do you see the leaf-cutter ants marching down the tree, carrying little pieces of leaves?" He pointed at the tree standing outside near the street.

I noticed the procession of ants moving down the tree trunk and along the ground and disappearing through a crack in the adobe wall. "Yes," I said, "I see them." And then he slid his foot across their path, disrupting the ants, sending them and the leaf fragments in all directions.

"Now what do you see?"

I watched as the ants searched frantically for their path, and then one and another found it and reconnected the line. In a few minutes, it was as if nothing had happened.

"Yes," I said, "I see."

"That is what happens all the time. The ants expect it to happen. They are not angry. They are not sad to lose a few pieces of leaf. They just want to find each other, to find their way again."

"But they're just ants. They don't know why they're doing this. It's just instinct. I need to understand why."

"It's the will of God," said Ricardo. "We are his servants, even if we do not understand his plan for us. I think you know what God has intended for you to do. You must do it."

And for a moment I could imagine my own grandfather talking to me. "Davidil," he'd say, "pray to God for forgiveness, for answers, for hope, and for strength. No one can understand all the reasons."

"I think I'll take a walk to the river," I said. I was not willing to imagine myself as an ant carrying a leaf, or Ricardo's foot as God, because then what was the point of it? And so I had to walk.

I walked down to where the swimming hole had been, but it was now a stagnant pool away from the main flow of the river. A flood five years before had altered the river's course away from the swimming hole. I crouched upon the gray granite rocks that used to provide shelter and a diving platform, and I gazed up the valley into the mountains. The rocks now served as a quiet refuge, a sanctuary for contemplation, which had been impossible among the noisy bathers.

Ricardo's words reverberated in my mind. "I would give up everything . . . I am happy . . . to rebuild our life better than it was before." That was why I had come back—to find that turn in the river, to retrace my steps, to start again. But the river had changed course, and the clinic was gone. The river now flowed faster and deeper, and a new clinic had replaced our clinic. Everything was different. Everything was fresh with new possibility.

I threw baseball-sized rocks along the riverbed—five, ten, twenty of them banging and clanging against the boulders, plopping into the water, sometimes skipping across the surface, and I imagined each one was something new that I could do. Then I balanced on the boulders and stepped from one to another. As I stepped from rock to rock, I created a path, but as I looked back, I knew I could never retrace it. I would touch different rocks, and I might even slip or fall on the rock that had held me securely before. My shoulders felt light, and my feet floated in the air as I hopped from one rock to the next, and I wondered why I had to come all the way back here to do this, why I couldn't do it at home. As I felt my breath fill my chest and the warmth of the sun on my face, I tried to be present in the moment, like the birds and cows, to appreciate the sounds and colors and smells around me and all the possibilities they presented. I felt a cool breeze brush softly over my face, like a hand. I peered out into the distance, following the green-gray contours of the mountains as they met the curves of the river. Cattle and burros fed by the river's edge, and a horse trail disappeared into the trees. A turkey vulture searching for animal remains among the rocks glided peacefully as it studied the earth from a distance. Other birds sang or sprinted across the river, but the vulture kept making long lazy loops up into the mountains.

Chapter Twenty-nine

"HOW WAS YOUR TRIP?" LAURA ASKED.

"Fine," I said. I had been back for only a day, and she had called to discuss the children.

We paused, each waiting for the other to talk.

"How were they, Ricardo and Rosa?" she finally asked.

"They're getting older. It's been hard," I said.

"What happened?"

"Tomás got kidnapped. They had to pay ransom. All of their money. Everything they owned, to get him back," I said.

"Did he make it?" she asked.

"Yes," I said.

"Thank God," she said. "There's nothing more precious than your children. I don't know what I would do if something happened to our kids."

I sighed. I wanted to say that what we were doing was hurting our children, and it made no sense. If they were so precious to her, why would she want to leave? But I just let the thought bounce around in my head and didn't let it out.

"Yes, I feel the same way," I said.

"What else did you do?" she asked.

"I walked around. I visited the clinic. I walked to the river and jumped over stones."

"Well, I'm glad you went there," she said.

"Yes, so am I."

"Now we have to make some plans. The kids will be coming home from camp. They will need some structure."

"I know," I said.

"It will be complicated. We'll need a schedule for each house, each day."

"You could come back," I said.

Laura's response was silence. I clutched my phone like a club, as if I could squeeze out a word like *yes* or *maybe*.

"No," she said.

"But you still love me," I said.

"How do you know?"

"Because I can feel it. And I love you too."

"If you love me, let me go," she said.

"But I do love you, and I don't want to let you go."

"If you love me, let me go."

"OK," I said. "If that's what I have to do. If that is what you want, I'll let you go."

"Thank you," she said.

I paused, waiting for her to say that she had reconsidered, but there was only another long silence. Then we talked about the kids again.

We talked about bills, schedules and trips, cars and food, computers and phone numbers, how many days each child would spend with each parent, how much money Laura would need, how we would tell parents and friends, and how to talk to our children. We talked about each detail as if we were discussing the weather, without emotion. I made a list, and we agreed to talk again in a few days.

When I put down the phone at the end of the conversation, my hand was sweaty, and my fingers twitched uncontrollably. My ear throbbed from the pressure of the telephone receiver as if some invisible foot had kicked me. I touched my earlobe and the cartilage with my fingers and then covered my ear with my palm, muffling all the sounds of the house in that ear. It was like putting my face underwater. When I moved my hand away, I was coming back to the surface.

I looked down at the list with the dates and activities and the responsible person, Mom or Dad. In the margins I had doodled the word *why*, extending the *y* into a long serpiginous river that followed a meandering course around the paper. Now I drew lines through the river, little dams creating segments where the river would back up into a cool pool of contemplation, where children might swim on a warm afternoon. And finally, I drew lines through the *w* and *h* and *y* and darkened them until the word was no longer legible and the river had lost its source and all that was left was the list with a pretty, decorative border.

I folded it into halves and then quarters, and as I placed the list in my upper left shirt pocket, my right hand came to rest there briefly.

It was an awkward place to touch, my beating heart just inches away. As a child I would put my hand there every day at the beginning of school as we stood and recited the pledge of allegiance. It would remind me of how powerful all of us could be together, with powerful hearts beating as one, voices pledging together. But now it reminded me of my patients who would indicate the location of the pain from a heart attack by putting a hand over the left part of the chest. How fragile and uncertain the heart could be. It could skip a beat and even stop. Then we would pound on it and shock it with electricity.

That's what we had to do to Mr. Harrison, my most recent patient to die of a heart attack. It was a few months ago, and he was laughing about the pain and joking about his previous heart attacks when he suddenly lay back in his bed, and the heart monitors sounded the alarms. He was surrounded by family, his wife, two daughters, four grandchildren. They called us when he fell back, and watched as we performed CPR.

"You did your best," said his wife, a small Chinese American woman with short gray hair. "I'm a nurse," she added. "We have been married for fifty years. We met during the war. We had a good life. I knew this would happen some day, but now that it has happened, I can't believe he's really gone. I don't know how to live without him."

I tried to listen, to help her accept it. Sometimes people ask whether we have a priest, what funeral home they should use, whether they can be with their loved ones alone, or why the death happened.

But if Mrs. Harrison had questions, she was holding them inside. I decided to provide answers to the questions I thought she might want to ask.

"He was old, and he seemed happy before he died. He did not suffer. He died suddenly with all of the people around him who loved him," I said.

His wife nodded. "Thank you."

Afterward I wondered if she would be one of those women who die shortly after their husbands die, because they could not bear to live without them. Or would she seize the new possibilities that life had suddenly given her? Would she join a gym, learn to play an instrument, find a new love?

As I touched my chest, I thought of Mr. and Mrs. Harrison, the pledge of allegiance, and my own heart and the list sitting in the pocket next to it. I thought of how difficult it was to let go of someone you loved, and I thought of the river—how it resembled a question mark as it meandered between the mountains, and how sometimes a river can change its course.

Epilogue

AFTER I RETURNED TO ALBUQUERQUE, I RESUMED MY WORK in the emergency department. Sometimes between patients I would ponder my visit. The turmoil in the village paralleled my own turmoil and put it in perspective. If the clinic could deteriorate, so could anything—a marriage, a friendship, a life. And it could also be reborn. Change was inevitable and not anyone's fault, and it made life frightening and exciting. The clinic's demise had prevented me from reliving many of the experiences that had propelled me into my career. But perhaps in reliving them, I would have created false memories to replace what was vague and fading. Instead, I had to rely upon the memories I had. Like the woman dying of tetanus or Ricardo's father dying of a stroke, my patients often arrived in that gray world between life and death. I wanted to be there for them, to either bring them back from the brink or help ease their passage into death. That's what I wanted to do for Mrs. Bitsitty, an elderly Navajo woman who arrived in the emergency department wearing a turquoise necklace over a maroon velvet blouse, and a red scarf over her silver hair. Mrs. Bitsitty was breathing in short gasps.

"Nezcash?" I attempted to ask about pain in Navajo.

She laughed at my clumsy attempt to speak her language. Even in pain, she could laugh.

"Nezcash," she said back to me and pointed to her chest.

I nodded. That would be the extent of my history unless we could find a Navajo interpreter, and at ten in the evening, that seemed unlikely. I had no old chart to detail any previous illnesses, though her identification tag indicated that she was eighty-seven years old. I ordered an EKG and called the internal medicine resident to admit her to the hospital.

The resident called me back on the telephone and asked me a succession of questions I could not answer.

"How long has she been in pain?" "Is the pain radiating to her arm?" "What are her cardiac enzymes?"

When I could not answer any of the questions, he asked me how I knew she needed to be admitted.

I couldn't explain it, but I just knew. Perhaps it was something in her facial expression, something in her breathing, but I knew.

A few hours later she went up to the intensive care unit. By then, her EKG had been done and was very suggestive of a heart attack. Within minutes of her arrival in the intensive care unit, Mrs. Bitsitty had a cardiac arrest and died.

Later that night, the internal medicine resident came down to the emergency department to tell me. I felt no satisfaction that my impression had been correct. I was only glad that I had been able to make her laugh before she died.

"How did you know?" the resident asked.

"I just knew," I said.

In the same way, I knew Carl would come back into my life. His absence during my visit to the clinic left me with a crucial gap in my quest for answers. I wanted to know what had happened since the scandal. And so I was not surprised when I heard that Carl was coming to Albuquerque to speak at a conference. I actually expected it, just as I had expected Mrs. Bitsitty to die. I decided to call him without any plan, curious to hear his voice and detect whether he had changed. He seemed pleased and genuine as we talked—his voice calm without any trace of agitation—and only mildly surprised at my call. I suggested we meet during the visit, expecting him to decline, to be too busy.

"Yes, I'd like that," he said, and we agreed upon a coffeehouse for our meeting.

From inside the coffeehouse, his twisted form, topped by a scraggly beard, was at once familiar and eerie. The streaks of gray in his hair and beard created a patchwork of color and contrast that camouflaged his facial features. Usually the lines in a face show up like skid marks on a road—markers of the tragedies or joys of life etched into the skin. But Carl's face, like his life, remained hidden.

"Well, you look good," I said.

"Thanks, but I've never looked good. Now I'm old enough to just look old."

"How's the clinic doing?"

"Not well. We've had to close. But Gabriel is there, and the government was so embarrassed by our previous success that they have opened a government clinic in the village."

"Yes, I was there. It was so sad to see the place like that."

"The entire village is in crisis. Drugs and violence have swept down from the mountains. Even the clinic was not immune from it."

"Do you think it will ever start up again?"

"I don't know. The times have changed. The needs have changed. Now we need a program to combat the violence. It's killing more people than tetanus, diarrhea, or tuberculosis."

"Yeah, I heard about Tomás when I visited Rosa and Ricardo. They told me you brought the money they needed."

"Well, I don't have much money left." He smiled. "That's why I come to conferences like this. They help pay the bills. But it's difficult to keep up the funding stream."

"Yeah, I heard about the newspaper story and the foundation."

"They don't understand anything. They destroy people just to sell newspapers. And the foundation is a bunch of cowards. Now, without me, it's nothing. Nothing."

"I still get their newsletter, but they seem to have lost direction," I said.

"*I* was their direction," he said and set his jaw.

"I heard about the allegations," I said. "The boys . . . I remember Luis, but I didn't know. He seemed very close to you."

"Thank you," he smiled. "I told them I never abused anyone. Every boy that I have ever known will confirm it. Abuse is about pain, neglect, hurt, and not caring. I have sent them through school, paid for medical care, listened to them, gone to their weddings, and become the godfather of their children. Was that wrong?"

"No."

"Love is not about an act. It's about caring and commitment to another human being. I am a teacher, and I teach what they want and need. Boys need attention at a certain age, and when you're with them all day and understand them the way I do, it is as natural as talking or eating. I have never forced anyone to do anything. Never. But I did try to be an important adult in their lives. A mentor. You knew that. I could tell you knew. The Greeks made relationships between boys and men a part of the culture and training. And what do we do? We throw our youth into the streets in gangs without any adults who care, and then recoil in horror at the violence. Am I a monster for caring about them?"

"No, but . . ."

"Look at me. Could I force anyone to do what he did not want to do? Look at my hands. Look at my face. What do you think?"

I scrutinized him. He had deep lines on his face and thin, translucent skin over his bony hands.

"But couldn't you have helped them and cared about them without . . ." I paused.

"Yes," he said. "And I did." He stared straight ahead, thinking. "They understood. They knew the truth. They have seen what we have done. The lives we've saved. Most of them are now doctors, dentists, and teachers, all because of me, you, the clinic. Because we care and give money or whatever we have for them."

"Why are you telling me this?"

"Because I want you to know. I don't want what we've built with our blood and sweat poisoned and ruined by people who don't understand. Because we must keep it alive and the spirit that built it alive. And that spirit was pure and good."

He paused, and I didn't know how to respond. I knew that what he had done was neither pure nor good, but that he would never recognize it, so I shifted into a more concrete realm.

"I saw Luis several years ago. He thinks you don't care about him. He was married and seemed to be doing well. But he seemed a little sad, and lost. I don't think your relationships are always positive for the boys. Sometimes I think they do get hurt."

"Yes, well I rarely ever meet boys anymore. And as for Luis, he knows that I do care for him. He just can't let go of me. He still wants me to tell him what to do. But I can't. Even though I think of him all the time, I won't do that to him. It wouldn't be fair." He paused and looked at me. "And what about you? How do you like Albuquerque?"

"Oh, it's fine. Albuquerque is becoming a big city with drugs and violence and traffic problems like everywhere else. And for me, it's . . . it's been difficult lately. My wife and I split up and . . ."

"Oh, I'm sorry to hear that."

"Yes, it's been difficult because we have two kids, teenagers. I worry about them. And I don't know what I could have done differently. But you need two people to make a marriage."

"Well, it seems that I hear these stories more and more. Couples married ten, twenty, thirty years decide to divorce. I suppose it's unnatural, living with the same person year after year, but I come to expect the stability of men and women in the same home, like a museum sculpture that never changes. One day I am a guest in their home and everything seems wonderful, and the next time I visit, they are separated. It's quite unsettling. Of course, I'd never venture a word of advice on this subject," he said.

"I used to look to you as a role model. I'd follow your activities through your newsletter. You were always devoted to the clinic, and you never worried about money."

"I worry about it now."

"Yes, but remember how everyone worked together—poor villagers, volunteers, landowners—and they made that clinic work."

"Well, it's not working now."

"I know, and that's what's so upsetting. It seems like everything is falling apart."

"Yes, but you know, babies are not dying of diarrhea or neonatal tetanus like when I first got to the village. We did solve that. They got clean water and immunizations. Now, there's the violence, but that's another kind of problem, and the clinic cannot solve it. At least not the old clinic. But you still have your children, your friends, and all the people that you save in the ER. How many lives do you think you've saved?"

"I don't know. In my whole life? Not that many. Every now and then, I'll save one that I think might have died if I hadn't been there."

"So, how many—five, ten, twenty, fifty?"

"Maybe twenty."

"So twenty people are alive who might not be if you hadn't been there. Not many people can say that."

"I guess so. But there are also lots of dead ones I didn't save. I didn't even know their names."

"But we are more than all the names of people we know. And the clinic was more than a place. The idea has spread. The idea that people without medical training can learn how to take care of themselves and their neighbors, and they don't need to sell their land to doctors or hospitals to get the medical care they need. That's an idea I share all over the world. That idea is alive and growing. And you can take an idea like that and make it into reality by coming back every day and working on it, believing in it. And soon others believe in it, all over the world."

"Yes, I've heard about your travels to India and China."

"It's funny how the idea has outlived the original creation. That's because when you have to take an idea and make it real, you have to make choices, and sometimes you make mistakes. Sometimes what you build has so many flaws that it all comes crumbling down. But the clinic lasted more than twenty-five years. And your marriage? How many years?"

"Sixteen. Sixteen years."

"And every day you had to make decisions and choices. They can't all be right. And at the same time, the world is changing around you. It's really quite an impossible task. But the idea is still there."

"I don't know," I said.

He paused, reflecting. "Well, when I realized the clinic would have to close, I blamed myself. I thought I had failed because I hadn't raised enough money or convinced enough people about what we needed to do. I had to let it go—or let go of the old picture—before I could envision a new one and appreciate all the things that had worked. I realized it was almost a miracle, what we did, with almost no money, just a few of us, volunteers and villagers. We had no idea what we were doing, and we made so many mistakes. But there was so much that grew out of it, just by our being there and giving. We created a place for people to come together, to make a connection with each other, to help each other at their most vulnerable moments, like lovers. That's why you keep thinking about it. That's why you go back again and again. But you won't find it there anymore; what's left of it is inside us."

"But don't you miss it?"

"All the time. I miss all of it, all of them. But I would do it all again— most of it, anyway. People told me the whole idea was crazy, and that it would never work. They were right that it was crazy, but it worked because I believed in it and you did and soon everyone did," he said.

We sat silently for a moment as I reflected on what he was saying.

"Yeah, when I got married, I thought I was crazy. I mean, here I was. I had never had any relationships that lasted for more than a year. We had been together for only eight months. We had no idea what we were getting ourselves into, but we believed in ourselves, and day by day we created a home and a family. But then we drifted apart. All the powerful forces that kept us together pushed us apart. Maybe it was miraculous that it lasted as long as it did."

"Yes, well, as I have said, I cannot give you any advice on marriage."

"And work seems meaningless. The same bloody faces and stab wounds day after day. What's the point?" I asked.

"The point is that you show up there day after day, and other people see you there, and you have created a place where people care, and a program where students learn and carry the idea forward. And if you are like me, the idea will grow and change and outlive the original four walls. But you must not confuse the place and the original idea with who you are now," he said.

It was a strange exchange, after so many years—each of us holding up his life for examination by the other, struggling to merge our images from the past with this brief moment, struggling for trust and acceptance. He put his hand on my shoulder for a moment before withdrawing it back onto his lap.

His hand was frail and small. I used to think of him as so much larger, a whirlwind of energy and ideas. Now I noticed all the debris around him. He was the man who had taught me about the exploitation of poor Mexican farmers, and he was the man who slept with the sons of those same farmers. All of his energy and money could not prevent the village from sinking into the muck and slime of kidnapping and violence. I wondered what his legacy would be, how we would remember him. Would it be the images of the clinic, the many people from the village whose lives had been changed, the Americans like me who returned to the United States to try to carry forward the same compassion and commitment to the poor that we had learned from him? Or would it be the scandal?

If my life had made a difference, I knew he had a hand in it. If my life had veered off, and I had lost the balance, perhaps the examples of his bad choices had steadied me.

"I need to go," I said, glancing at my watch.

"So do I," he said. And he walked out the door, creating a storm of dust particles in the reflected sunlight.

I returned to the hospital and walked through the emergency department. Rick was there with a harried look on his face.

"It's a seven-hour wait," he said.

"I'll see a few," I offered.

"Thanks. I owe you."

"No, remember the Mexico shifts."

"Oh, yeah," he said. "You owe *me*."

"I just saw that guy, Carl. He's here in Albuquerque."

"Did he try to goose you?" Rick asked.

"Rick, what?" I asked.

"Well, I mean, since you've started running again and lost a few pounds, I was, you know, a little worried."

"Rick, forget it. I'm not going to help you," I said.

"Oh, come on. I was just pulling your chain," he said.

The nurses asked me to see a patient with a laceration. He was a carpenter who had cut his hand when he fell from a ladder. They were exasperated, and the patient had waited a long time.

"Sure," I said, and I put on gloves to explore the wound.

It was a simple cut, and the man was in a hurry. I looked into the wound past the skin and blood, deeper into the wound where the nerves and tendons lay hidden near the bones. Even though I knew I would find everything intact, I exposed the wound, as always, to know for sure that there was nothing else wrong. And this time, as my mind drifted to my conversation with Carl, I probed absently into the wound and felt something gritty and hard that should not have been there—a piece of glass.

"You have a piece of glass in your wound," I said. "How'd that happen?"

"Damned if I know," he said. "I guess it was on the ground."

I removed the sharp glass fragment and lay it on the instrument tray. It had a triangular shape with blood around the edges.

"Here it is," I said and showed him.

"Damn, that's ugly," he said.

I had been admiring the sparkles and contours, the red outline and the surprise of it. I nodded. I knew what he meant.